American
Shamans

Also from **Busca**

Healing of the Soul: Shamanism and Psyche

Universal Kabbalah: Dawn of a New Consciousness

Battlegrounds of Freedom: A Historical Guide to the
Battlefields of the War of American Independence

Devil Dogs and Jarheads

A Farm Girl in the Great Depression

American Shamans

Journeys with Traditional Healers

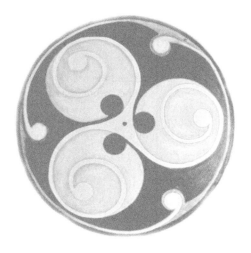

JACK MONTGOMERY

BuscaInc.

Ithaca, New York

Busca, Inc.
5930 Route 414, Hector, NY 14841
PO Box 854, Ithaca, NY 14851
www.buscainc.com
Telephone: 607-546-4247; Fax: 607-546-4248

Copyright © 2008 Jack Montgomery
First Edition

American edition printed in the United States of America.

Any references to healing practices are intended as general information rather than substitutions for professional medical and therapeutic consultations.

Publisher's Cataloging-In-Publication Data

(Prepared by The Donohue Group, Inc.)

Montgomery, Jack G.

  American shamans : journeys with traditional healers / Jack Montgomery.

    p. ; cm.

  Includes bibliographical references.

  ISBN-13: 978-0-9666196-9-0

  ISBN-10: 0-9666196-9-2

1. Shamanism--United States. 2. Spiritual healing--United States. 3. Traditional medicine--United States. I. Title.

BL2370.S5 M66 2008

299/.4

Book design and composition: Paperwork

Cover art: *Triskele in Ochres* by Christina Scurr. Hand-painted shaman drum, 16.5 inches, semi-transparent hide on beech frame with oil paint. Available from Drum Spirit: Hand Painted drums by Christina Scurr at *www.drumspirit.co.uk/shamen.htm*. Reproduced here through the generous courtesy of the artist.

Contents

Acknowledgements

I WOULD LIKE TO THANK all the people who made this book possible. First, my principal contacts: James E. McTeer, Lee Raus Gandee, "Sarah Ramsey," "Oracle," "Rose," Granny Harmon and everyone else who generously shared their thoughts and experiences with me over the years. I appreciate Catherine Yronwode's insights on Hoodoo. I am grateful to Dr. Saundra Ardrey, Department Head of Political Science and Director of the African American Studies Program at Western Kentucky University, for her review of Chapter One and for sharing her personal story of healing. My sincere thanks go to the Reference librarians at the Beaufort County (South Carolina) Public Library, Fran Hays, Rachel Kingcaid and Grace Morris Cordial, for their generous help in researching articles on Mr. McTeer.

Elizabeth Hayes helped me greatly with her editorial review of Chapter One, and her spiritual insights were much appreciated. I would especially like to thank Roxanne Myers Spencer for her invaluable editorial skills and steadfast commitment to helping me with the entire book; your considerable efforts helped make this book all that it could be.

I would like to thank my dear wife Lesley for her infinite patience while I labored nights, weekends and holidays on this project. I will make it up to you somehow. Thanks also to all my friends for your input and comments. No one can do something like this in a vacuum.

Finally, I would like to thank that Divine presence that pervades everything for inspiring me to write this memoir and for giving me a reason to exist. You are, in the final analysis, the only real magic.

Why Write this Book?

The most beautiful thing we can experience is the mysterious. It is the source of all true art and all science. He to whom this emotion is a stranger, who can no longer pause to wonder and stand rapt in awe, is as good as dead: his eyes are closed.
—Albert Einstein, (1879–1955)

All we know is still infinitely less than all that remains unknown.
—Willaim Harvey, (1578–1657)

THIS BOOK has taken thirty years to write. Not because of the length of the research, although that continues to this day. I began this journey of the mind and spirit as a college student looking for a novel topic on which to research. I had to write a single term paper in comparative religion. My major was religious studies with a minor in psychology and significant coursework in anthropology.

It was through reading ethnographies that I became fascinated with the idea of actually going into a community and studying the relationships and dynamics. I continue to be interested in community beliefs, systems, ideas and concepts that develop outside formal educational and religious institutions. The common knowledge, the knowledge passed from parent to child, sibling to sibling and throughout the greater community, fascinates me personally and intellectually. This community wisdom, the shared experiences and ways of conducting one's life forms an intimate, often unconscious, base on which all our education rests. This background becomes a filter through which we view and construct our realities.

Today, community folklore and folk beliefs are most often studied academically in colleges and universities. Students and others may be drawn to these subjects when modern conceptions of reality and the imposed structures of rationality affect our psychological existence and are inadequate to meet our basic human spiritual needs. These spiritual needs are strongest during the major events in our lives: birth, love, illness, madness, danger and death. These are the times when we seek answers beyond those offered by our modern humanistic and rationalistic society. A quest for understanding our existence reaches beyond the realms of the vicarious existence perpetrated through the popular media as part of the information-driven, postindustrial society we live in.

In dire circumstances, such as a child stricken with an inexplicable illness, parents may not merely want to hear about probabilities of recovery. There is little comfort in the strictly biological facts. For this reason, most hospitals provide a chapel or a chaplain, to offset the sterility of laboratories and lonely waiting rooms. In a strictly rational sense, a chaplain and a hospital chapel should not be able to provide any comfort, yet they often do. Modern scientific studies have also shown that the seemingly meaningless words and acts of these virtual strangers seem to provide some aid to the patient as well, allowing for an enhanced sense of well being and even accelerated recovery.

We might ask ourselves what possible good it could do to have someone lay their hands on a patient and recite old-fashioned prayers from days long past. Yet a laying-on of hands often provides comfort in physical, psychological and spiritual cases when it is applied. What is this person doing? Where did this arcane practice come from?

These kinds of questions led me to a fascination with the non-medical healer in our society. This is the person who addresses our physical and emotional needs, helps us answer questions and resolve conflicts and often helps us prepare for the unknown future. They can, in some cases, reach beyond the mundane and help us deal with what appear to be unseen forces that motivate and direct our lives.

Modern anthropology referred to this type of person in earlier times as a shaman, the person in a community who performed rituals associated with healing, with interpretation of events, who might predict future events and who envisioned our role in those events. As I studied and researched this diverse topic, I realized that although we may call them by different names, there are still many individuals performing in a shamanic manner in our society today. I also realized that there were still people operating in our cities and communities in an older, more traditional role of shaman. I set out to find and learn what I could about and from these people.

What started as an interesting undergraduate paper for a religious studies class at the University of South Carolina (USC) in the mid-1970s became a quest for knowledge, heritage and personal meaning. This journey took me to places I would have never visited otherwise. It placed me in contact with some truly special people that changed and enhanced the quality of my life forever. As I look back, I am amused at my own brashness and naiveté. I would take off fearlessly into the back roads of rural South Carolina with notepad, tape recorder and camera, determined to discover the unknown and the miraculous. The Bible reminds us that you will find that which you seek. That certainly was the case with me, although I was not always prepared for what I found.

This book is, therefore, a memoir of my experiences with several American shamanic healers. My mother has a saying, "There are many worlds within this world of ours." She is referring, of course, to the many cultures that make up the patchwork quality of American culture. She is also referring to the different perceptions and conceptions of reality that exist side by side in what should be a modern, media-induced social homogeny. Cultural beliefs and practices persist despite attempts to ridicule and otherwise eliminate them. The truth is that those folk beliefs, mythic structures, ritualized behaviors, superstitions and other practices provide us with personal and social identity, mental equipoise and a sense of focus and purpose to cope with the events and people we encounter.

Modern discoveries of quantum mechanics and string theory reveal that, at a certain level of atomic existence, the laws of modern physics do not seem to work in a rational manner. The human psyche also often does not react the way it is trained or expected to behave. There is, at that deep level, another dynamic at play that cannot be refuted. Much like the quark in astrophysics, we know it is there by its effect on things and events we can measure. The science and study of modern psychology and human consciousness are only about 100 years old; hence, we have much to learn about the abilities and potential of the human mind.

One of the other reasons it has taken me thirty years to tell this story was a hesitation and uncertainty of how to present these unusual events. I have spent many years trying to interpret them, explain them away and otherwise dismiss their value. I will refer to events that occurred during my research which seem, at some level, strange and miraculous to the average reader.

I also wanted to avoid the ridicule and disdain of those who cannot cope with, and subsequently fear, the presence of things beyond their conventional reality and who will invariably attack the messenger for attempting to discuss them. To those folks, I can offer no comfort in their dilemma; they must perceive and process what I relate here through their own lens on reality.

As a result, I have decided to present these unusual events as I personally experienced them, at that time, without embellishment. Even so, some of you may decide that such things are absurd and dismiss this book and me as a result. I suspect, however, that those readers who have experienced the unusual, the mystical or the miraculous in their lives may hear a familiar voice in my writings.

Recently, I was having a conversation with a friend regarding biblical miracles and their meaning to our society today. He was busily explaining how these events really were not miracles, but that the people and chroniclers involved simply did not know how else to interpret their experience. I asked him if he thought it was possible for people today to experience miracles or whether it was simply a matter of proper interpretation. He thought for a moment and said, "I don't actually know, but I'd like to think it is still possible."

Like my friend, I firmly believe in the progress and advances of modern science and objective review of our experiences. Yet I also wish to retain an open mind to the possibility of the miraculous.

After the experiences I relate in this book, I eventually wrote and presented several lectures to university classes, civic and religious groups and taught a short course on the topic, as part of University of South Carolina's Free University program. The formal paper was submitted in 1976 as a senior thesis for a baccalaureate degree, and I supposed that was an end to the matter. At the time, I believed my grand adventure into academic fieldwork had ended; yet it had only just begun. All these years later, it is still a grand adventure that I hope to share with you in the pages of this book.

Several years ago, I was riding a train through western Pennsylvania on my way to visit friends in Indiana. Across the aisle from me sat a well-dressed young woman who was very pregnant and seemed uncomfortable by the motion of the train. I was unable to sleep, also because of the motion of the train, so we began talking quietly. She lived in Pittsburgh, and her husband worked in a factory. She had wanted to finish school but the impending arrival of her baby had suspended her college education. Somehow, in the conversation, I mentioned an interest in folk religion and my hope of finding some local sources while visiting my friends. I told her of my background research into Pennsylvania folk religion and the practice of Powwowing.

"Oh," she replied, "I know about that! I remember that throughout my childhood, when I would get sick, my mother or dad would go for the Powwow doctor. He would stand over me and say something in German. I never understood it, but I always seemed to get better right away."

I asked her if she believed in Powwows now, and with a grin, she replied, "Well, not until I get sick!"

This comment seems to contradict a statement made 100 years ago in the *Popular Science Monthly* article "Magical Medical Practice in South Carolina," by South Carolina historian, John Hawkins, that such beliefs:

> . . . yield almost imperceptibly to the advance of sound learning and com-
> mon sense. Their retreat, however, has been more rapid since science
> has begun to shed her ray into the dark places where such things hide
> themselves; and in proportion as this great light becomes more genuinely
> diffused, magic in medicine, as in all other departments of human thought,
> will fade away and finally disappear. (174)

During the past thirty years, I have come to realize just how presumptu-ous Mr. Hawkins' statement was and still is today. The beliefs, far from fading away with the advancement of science, have remained, although, in some instances, they have retreated to the more rural areas of our great nation and into the "dark places" of what we now refer to as the subconscious mind. Far from fading into the electronic oblivion of our postindustrial society, even the casual observer cannot help but notice that the "Old Arts" of astrology, faith healing, mysticism and witchcraft have experienced a renaissance, powered and transmitted by that most modern of tools, the Internet.

The viability and persistence of these seemingly archaic beliefs seem to be confirmed by the comments of the young mother in Pennsylvania noted above, and also by an old shopkeeper who ran a grocery store in a small community near Beaufort, South Carolina. The shopkeeper once said to me, "Son, you can't possibly think that people went to the moon in 1969? The moon is a magical entity and no man can ever touch it. What the astronauts did was to go out in the desert and make-believe on TV that they went to the moon so as to fool us—but everybody knows better."

However irrational and unscientific such remarks may appear, there exists and persists in this day an almost incalculable measure of the ancient and primitive, symbolically riding its broomstick alongside the astronaut into the twenty-first century. To try to deny or dismiss its existence and continued impact on our culture is understandable but also somewhat narrow and vain. The man from Beaufort asserted his disbelief in the physical existence of the moon, which to him was within the realm of another reality. Are we not doing the same, based on our beliefs, as well?

This book is also the recollection of a journey into that other world of perception and belief that continues to co-exist with its modern scientific counterpart. We can attempt to flee from this split within ourselves of the rational and the inexplicable. It can become a tormentor from which we frantically and futilely try to escape, as did the main character in Guy de Maupassant's classic 1887 tale, *The Horla*; yet it will continue, like a menacing shadow, to chase us. On the other hand, we can journey along with this mysterious shadow, much as we do with our physical shadow, perceiving it as an integral part of our being, and giving it the respect it deserves. Only then will we be left undisturbed, intellectually and personally, by its presence and be able to learn the lessons it may have to share with us.

Beginning the Fieldwork: Finding My Primary Contacts

Three of the primary field-research contacts are deceased, and the others have asked that their actual names not be used. I intend, as much as possible, to let their words speak for themselves and to treat the memory of those now gone with the respect, patience and kindness they extended to me. I will provide some additional background on the history and culture of my contacts, and I will offer my own observations and insights gleaned over the years. I am relying on my written notes, taped interviews, scholarly supportive materials and my memories to tell this story. I hope the reader will gain insight into and an understanding of the special people who lived and, in a sense continue to live, as their traditions live on.

A friend, reading this manuscript, asked me how I initially located my contacts. As I began to read and research these topics in the region of the Carolinas, I would occasionally find, as I did with Lee Raus Gandee, an article in a local magazine, which led me to his door. The same situation occurred with J. E. McTeer; after being alerted to his existence by a college friend, an article in a newspaper led me to seek him out.

I contacted the person I will call "Granny Ramsey" through personal referrals from her granddaughter. Her story can be told while protecting the family's privacy. Unlike J. E. McTeer and Lee Gandee, Granny Ramsey had never been public with her abilities, nor had anything written about her. She came from a small rural Virginia community that has, as many Southern communities do, a desire to present themselves as free from super-stition and in line with their current conservative Christian sentiments. As her daughter pointed out to me, "You can leave and go home, but we have to live here and live with whatever you write about Momma." I intend to honor her wishes to be anonymous and hope the reader understands my protecting her identity. Hers is a story, like the others, that should be told, and her actual identity does not add or detract from it. In reality, each of these people reflects elements of their particular cultural background. Each has a worldview that is shared with others in their community to varying degrees of intensity.

The Structure of this Book

1. I will endeavor to present the people and events within the context of their historical, social and psychological settings. I cannot hope to cover the entire range of the history or all the social factors that affected these people and communities, but I will try to provide the reader with some ambience of the time. I will also offer short biog-raphies of my principal contacts, followed by selected transcripts of

my interviews and recollections of my encounters.

2. I wish to state from the outset that few clear distinctions exist between the practices of the root doctor, Powwow or granny-woman in terms of unique cultural elements. In every case, there is ample evidence of each of these traditions sharing ideas, concepts and practices. There are, therefore, no ethnically or racially pure expressions of these traditions, such as might be found in some remote jungle or island. Even the geographical divisions I've drawn in South Carolina reflect only the general locale of the tradition and a concentration of certain beliefs and practices.

3. I also have made the conscious choice to not to attempt to report the interviews in their original regional dialects. Focusing on accents, I believe, detracts from the central theme of communicating ideas and concepts.

4. In terms of subject content, this book is primarily focused on the magical practices of these communities. It does not deal in any depth the use of herbs and food remedies, even though the use of herbs is an important component of all three traditions, root doctor, Powwow and granny-woman. I've chosen to focus on the magical aspects because they are often neglected in this sort of study.

5. One particular reason I sought and still seek the input and counsel of living practitioners of these traditions is to honor the survival of these subtle, spiritual traditions. By recognizing that even though culturally jumbled, these practices are alive, and living people have something to add to the body of accepted knowledge on the subject. I also want to avoid the trap into which many who study esoteric traditions in academia unconsciously slip: the trap of publications as reliance for authority. Myshele Goldberg, doctoral student, wrote in the *PanGaia* article, "What's in a Name? Colonial Dynamics in Spiritual Practice":

Insisting on books as cultural "authorities" rather than honoring living tradition-bearers spotlights a common pattern of colonizers everywhere: to take oppressors' word over the word of indigenous people, even where tradition and folklore are concerned. This pattern manifests in anthropology, spirituality, and even activism, where the vast majority of literature is written by members of dominant groups. The underlying assumption is that living traditions no longer exist, or that they are somehow less "pure" than the material in books.

Living traditions can never be "pure." Like good friendships and healthy ecosystems, they are messy and full of contradictions, in a state of dynamic equilibrium. Static "purity" can come only at the price of cultural genocide, once traditions have been confined to history books. For a colonizer, that is where they belong. For a colonizer, history books are naturally the answer to nostalgia for "the old ways." By poaching traditions from the pages of books, a member of the colonizing class can avoid facing both his ancestors' actions and the survivors' grandchildren. Consulting books is much safer than consulting real people, and the power relationship is much closer to one a colonizer has grown accustomed to: books can be easily dismissed or selectively read. Real people can't always be silenced when their memories become uncomfortable. (23)

In the Western academic-intellectual tradition, which has followed and, to some degree, rationalized the political and cultural domination of other cultures, the written record reflects the cultural bias and parental attitude toward those most like themselves. In fact, academics, like those immersed in the world of high fashion, often "dress for each other" and for the approval of their particular group of peers. Such peer-groups often develop a tribal-like clique-ishness. Those who wish to be admitted or accepted must conform to the dominant ideas and standards of the clique or face rejection and censure until they can vindicate themselves. This form of domination can provide for a uniform response from the group at the price of innovative thinking and expression.

A classic case of this sort of group-stance is found Katherine Mayo's 1927 book on Hindu society, *Mother India*. Written from the standpoint of the British colonial system and the missionary efforts of the Christian churches, every native religious tradition, every social custom, was derided, lampooned and dismissed within its pages. Sadly, the views expressed in this tome and others like it formed the lens through which Hindu culture was perceived by the West many for several generations to come. The fact that this type of political and ethnocentric bias was tolerated reflects the social history of the period, yet its enduring damage to the perception of Hindu culture remains. I suppose nothing can be done to stop these sorts of offenses, except that we need to be aware of and sensitive to the fact that we all carry certain cultural biases. We cannot allow them to block or inhibit our perceptions when examining new or different practices and cultures. I believe that if we can initially keep an open mind to that which is new to us, the journey that we make through life will be richer and more rewarding.

I hope the reader finds this journey as fascinating as I did. I bid you welcome to a worldview that is perhaps very different from your own. Please try to proceed with an open mind, and you will receive the most from this personal memoir.

—JACK MONTGOMERY
AUTUMN 2007

What Is Magic? What Are Magical Healings and Shamanism?

My own suspicion is that the universe is not only queerer than we suppose, but queerer than we can suppose.

—J. B. S. Haldane, *Possible Worlds and Other Essays*, 1927

There is something in the human spirit that resists the idea of limits. . . . Things we once believed were magical and beyond the realm of possibility . . . are now considered normal.

—Lee Raus Gandee, (1917–1998), *Hexenmeister*

LET US BEGIN WITH THE CONCEPT OF MAGIC.

In this age of the Internet, the quark, virtual reality and the nanosecond, it seems nostalgic and quaint to even consider a concept like magic and absurd to apply it to the idea of healing. With all the many types of medical therapies and remedies currently available, why should any rational, modern person consider a non-scientific one?

If we have a stomachache or some easily identifiable distress, we can quickly turn to the vast array of potions and preparations prepared for us by modern drug companies for universal consumption. We reach for these remedies because we have been assured by personal experience and the relentless indoctrination of the mass media that they are safe and effective. In doing so, we assume these preparations have been tested and authenticated by scientific research, so we can all feel confident taking these unknown substances for relief, even though they may not always work as intended or have negative side effects.

To most of our recent ancestors, however, such a blind trust in impersonal pharmaceutical companies would seem an incredible leap of faith and even somewhat foolish. To many of our ancestors, removing the idea of Divine intervention or some power beyond ourselves from the healing process would seem just as outrageous as the way we now view our ancestors' reliance on non-scientific factors.

Today, if we are depressed, nervous or otherwise emotionally troubled, we have an army of mental health professionals to provide counsel and mind-altering medications, if necessary, to restore our sense of well-being, all based in the scientific/secular human worldview. This new professional class has publicly replaced the role once filled by pastor, priest, guru or shaman, relegating them and the beliefs they once espoused, to a quaint subclass of cultural advisor.

I am not attacking the use of scientific medicine or psychological therapies; I am simply trying to illustrate the basic difference between the current scientific worldview of healing and health and its older, but still living ancestor. I am not passing judgment on either system but want to make the reader aware of how quickly one system can appear to dominate the other publicly and politically. Those other systems, however, appear to survive in spite of the relentless indoctrination and derision by the dominant culture.

Author and sociologist James McClenon, in his essay, "Supernatural Experience, Folk Beliefs and Spiritual Healing," explains the problem of science and the supernatural:

> The concept of the supernatural has been shaped by the Western notion of nature and causality. Science has evolved in a manner that is restrictive and sometimes dysfunctional when applied to the supernatural. . . . Science focuses on "nature," a domain subject to empirical investigation. It tends to ignore the "supernatural," an area whose existence is uncertain. (108)

It is relevant to note that time has passed quickly in terms of the amount and degree of cultural change in the last one hundred years. The scientific, rational view of reality has superimposed itself over traditional belief systems that have been in place for thousands of years. The emergence of psychology as an accepted method of interpreting human experience is one example of this rapid change. Author and scholar David J. Hufford relates how:

> In the twentieth century, the Freudian psychoanalytic theory—an enormously popular belief system that has affected every aspect of American

intellectual life—identified all spiritual belief as a neurotic defense mechanism, an illusion based on infantile wish-fulfillment. (24)

For example, we are seeing a small, but determined cultural backlash against the purely scientific worldview with the arguments regarding human origins put forward by the Creationists. I suspect that science and evolution as concepts are not the problem. The problem, as I see it, lies in the arrogance and intolerance of other views by those who are possessed of limited vision, regardless of their educational background. Assertions of scientific rationalism and dogmatic intolerance still have quite a way to go in allowing for basic diplomacy and coexistence with other worldviews.

In fairness, during the last twenty years, the science-based medical community has begun to recognize the value of such practices as prayer, meditation and spiritual belief in the healing process. Our recent ancestors would be proud of them for their wisdom in looking back for inspiration.

The Idea of Magic

To be able to examine magical healing as a practice, we need to define what we mean by the word magic. German ethnologist and psychologist, Holger Kalweit, in his book, *Shamans, Healers and Medicine Men,* describes magic as:

> . . . neither a cultural fantasy of primitive people nor a complex of symbols and metaphors; rather, it is the natural means of exploration of a much more complex structure of consciousness than that currently used by the modern sciences in their exploration of reality. Magic is not below our present level of knowledge but beyond it. Magic is a state of cognition that psychology has yet to attain. (189)

Kalweit goes on to assert that the influence and position of magic in the development of Western European culture is considerable and pervades much of the history of our intellectual and religious development.

Any student of anthropology will immediately recognize the many magical practices that are prevalent in our Judeo-Christian religious traditions. Despite assertions to the contrary, magic and religion are often intertwined or overlap in ritual practices and ideas. One of the most familiar magical acts known is the invocation of a Divine or supernatural presence and the expression of an appeal for assistance or guidance. That appeal is followed by an expression of gratitude and by ritually closing with the magical word of closure: Amen.

We call this form of spiritual communication a prayer. The Catholic tradition often follows a more formal ritual appeal, called a novena. We often employ ritual items such as symbols (rosaries, prayer shawls, etc.) and may wear ritual garments, such as priestly robes, or head coverings to enhance our experience. We often engage in ritual speech and gestures, such as the holding together of our palms, kneeling, chanting or singing. We may sometimes engage in shamanic behavior, such as speaking in tongues, ecstatic dance or movement, all of which are rooted in a distant magical past.

An excellent example of this magically based behavior is the symbolic cannibalism found in the Christian ritual of Holy Communion. In its earliest, non-Christian form, this ritual was originally designed to magically imbue the worshipper with the traits and presence of Jesus, now described in the Bible as an act of remembrance.

The ancient ritual of first honoring, then torturing and finally slaying the chosen one or king, as a scapegoat for human sins was one well known to the ancient peoples of Europe and the Middle East. In many cases, the sacrificed body, now a symbol of holiness, was publicly displayed, consumed or taken home in pieces to bless the fields or hearth.

In many of these cultures, this human or animal symbol would rise again, to become the next designated sacrifice the following spring, as a symbolic promise of the return of the earth's fertility and the blessing of forgiveness. The acts of identification with and consuming of the sacrifice was designed to magically create a bond between the worshipper and the Divine, although, today, people may or may not immediately recognize this act for what it is.

I still remember, as a senior in college, giving a talk in a local Baptist church about cults and magical practices. I attempted to draw a parallel between the trance behaviors of Voodoo to that of the Christian Pentecostal ritual of speaking in tongues, which I had observed in my fieldwork. As you might imagine, several people in the congregation took personal exception to my comment, insisting that the two expressions could not be similar. They felt I was attacking their cherished beliefs, which they saw as the only correct views. After restoring a measure of calm, I assured them I was not assaulting the uniqueness of their particular beliefs, and then I finished my talk. As I left, the minister privately confided in me that he shared my conclusions but also knew many of his parishioners "were just not ready to hear" or to acknowledge the similarity of experience. His comments, voiced to me in this manner, reveal the ambiguous situation in which many priests, pastors and even academic scholars find themselves when trying to examine and interpret spiritual topics and issues to their audiences. While trying to maintain their public image as a rational, modern person, they often struggle with ideas that, by their nature, live outside the current range of socially acceptable beliefs and behaviors. Folklorist and author Erika Brady adds:

> Whether by vocation or profession, it appears that all—priests, folklorists, or professional pundits—who undertake to interpret the nature of human belief in the supernatural, place themselves willy-nilly in the role of umpires of the empirical, whether or not they claim such authority. (155)

This story illustrates the sensitive nature of such ideas and beliefs, and the often-imperceptible manner in which they are internalized as a part of our culture and life experience. I found, interestingly, that many of my informants in the field had similarly uncritically internalized the validity of magic and the reality of the supernatural in their lives.

In our modern popular culture, magically based beliefs appear to go in and out of popular acknowledgment as acceptable, or even fashionable. Faith-based healing, an inherently magical practice, was once overtly and then subtly ridiculed by the scientific, medical and academic intelligentsia as well as the media, but is now enjoying a revival of public expression in modern evangelical Christianity.

As *Hexenmeister* Lee Raus Gandee once said, "There is something in the human spirit that resists the idea of limits. . . . Things we once believed were magical and beyond the realm of possibility, such as space travel and organ transplants are now considered normal."

The Esoteric Dynamic of Magic

Magic, as we will see in the interviews later in this book, is considered the acquisition, accumulation, manipulation and projection of Divine or human energy. We must consider—from the magical and shamanic worldview—that this energy is, like the Divine, omnipresent. It exists everywhere and in everything to varying degrees of intensity. This includes inanimate and animate objects and the atmosphere itself. The universe, from the magical view, is an immeasurably vast, but finite living entity or field of energy. We exist, from this perspective, in an aquarium-like environment. Therefore, within this closed space we can draw energy into ourselves and send it out again, much as fish breathe by taking and expelling water through their gills. Similar to the way we take in food, water and air, all conscious entities can absorb psychic energy from our environment to be able to nourish our mental, spiritual and emotional capacities.

In such a universe, there are no random events, no accidents, with all events originating from a source somewhere within this sphere of energy. To act magically is to consciously gather, manipulate and then direct that energy toward a desired objective. By this definition, magical acts are simply enhanced versions of very normal processes of thought and action. By the same token, we can also recognize subtle cues as to distant and possible future events in our own sphere, which may directly affect us. The honing of this ability is how most healers and shamans are adept at sensing and interpreting what are popularly called signs or omens. These omens can be overt physical manifestations of the subtle movement of energy, such as the appearance of a certain animal or simply a change in the weather. These omens or signs can also be sensed psychically by those trained to seek and recognize their presence. This divination, or subtle sensing, might include entities or spirits that do not have a physical form dense enough to be detected by our usual five senses.

To illustrate this point, I brought my former college roommate, whom I will call "Gary," with me during one of my interviews with Powwow Lee Gandee. I wanted Gary to observe the situation and give me feedback on the people and events. Gary relayed to Lee an account of a psychic experiment involving astral travel. In this experiment, Gary attempted to project his image from one room to another, where his brother was ready to receive an agreed-upon sign, where Gary held up a certain number of fingers. Upon awakening, Gary asked his brother how many fingers he'd seen, and the brother reported the correct number. Gary was still curious about what had happened and asked Lee for insight into the phenomenon.

LG: Well, it's a complicated thing. It sounds like the same sort of process that goes on when you start dreaming. That is, the disassociation of the two levels of the mind. As long as your conscious mind is hooked in enough to hold your subconscious or the unconscious, it remains stable, or natural, just like you are now. You won't be able to see any of those things, but as you relinquish parts of it, it doesn't go all at one time. It goes piecemeal, and it concentrates on what you are trying to get it to concentrate on somewhere else. You may not see more than a suggestion of it because it's not perception in the sense of seeing objects that we see outside. They're hardly anything real, either. They're just constructs. But they're alive and they're part of it. The other kind are not. But, in handling these things, you very often see the essence of them rather than the substance, which is something you don't do in the other consciousness—the sensory version of the mind. Not like the consciousness without the senses. Does that make any sense to you?

Gary: No, it doesn't.

JM: You need to clarify that for Gary.

LG: I mean, if you could imagine yourself feeling something without a hand, without fingers to feel with. You could just imagine yourself as palming something. Well, you can do it if you think of certain textures. If you had a pair of corduroy pants or corduroy coat that you have worn for a long time, you don't have to touch the corduroy to feel it, do you?

Gary: I understand.

LG: Well, when you are feeling with that kind of consciousness—that you can get the sensation of feeling corduroy without touching it with your fingers—that's the difference between what I'm talking about as feeling with your consciousness and feeling with your sensors.

A shaman must also be able to sense the presence of concentrated energy within the natural physical environment, respond effectively to and manipulate it. Many shamans practice a form of geomancy and can draw energy from special sources found within the natural environment. These areas are sometimes referred to as places of power, vortexes and sacred spaces. Most of us have experienced the feeling of relaxation and well-being while sitting by a stream or standing atop a mountain. The shaman's experience is a more intense version of these feelings and can involve, at times, the need to interact with the consciousness of such a place. The consciousness of place is called an elemental. In a universe composed of various forms of concentrated energy, it is viewed in the shamanic perspective as only natural that some of these concentrations would develop a form of self-awareness. In the past, humans have devised many names and descriptions of these entities, including angels, devils, faeries, elves and ghosts.

But Is the Practice of Magic Religious?

One cannot and should not ignore the religious and spiritual side of these types of shamanic or magical practice. Certainly, our ancestors did not make such a distinction. Many of them consciously practiced some form of folk religion as an integral part of, or as an enhancement to, their faith. Folklorist Don Yoder, in the *Western Folklore* article "Toward a Definition of Folk Religion," traces the idea of folk religion to Germany at the turn of the last century when Lutheran seminary students needed a way to "better deal with the people in their rural congregations, whose conception of the Christian Religion was often radically different from the official doctrinal versions represented by the clergy" (3).

Scholars had defined this body of beliefs and practices in European culture from "survivals in the present of pre-Christian forms of religion" to "a mixture (the mélange) of an official 'high' religion with 'native' or 'primitive' religion" to a cultural "fringe phenomena in religion" to the "totality of all those views and practices of religion that exist among the people apart and alongside the strictly theological and liturgical forms of official religion" (Yoder 12-14).

There are many ways to view these cultural phenomena. As we will see in the following chapters, the idea of a belief system socially separate and yet coexisting with those of the dominant culture, are understandable, and to some degree justifiable, in light of the historical context in which they developed. It will also become clear that the survival of these belief systems was often due to the social neglect and the disenfranchisement of various groups of people within the greater American society.

On a more positive note, a similar case can be made that the survival of these same beliefs has added to and positively enhanced the cultural richness and diversity of American society. The persistence of these beliefs illustrates the patchwork quality of our heritage; these diverse beliefs have been stitched together to form a rich, yet distinctly American culture.

Let us now examine the basic concept of shamanism.

What Is a Shaman?

Roger Walsh offers a broad definition of shamanism in his book, *The Spirit of Shamanism,* which examines the subject from the perspective of modern psychology. A shaman, in this context, refers to persons "who enter controlled alternate states of consciousness, no matter which alternate states these may be" (6).

Historian and author Miranda Aldhouse-Green says in *The Quest for the Shaman,* that the word shaman "is a Siberian Tungus word and simply means 'ecstatic one'" (10). Green adds, "Shamanism is not even a religion as such but rather a worldview system or a grammar of the mind" (10).

Ethnologist Holger Kalweit states that in many of the world's traditions, shamans were often mythical and considered "identical with the founders of culture" (*Shamans, Healers* 9).

Anthropologist Michael Harner, founder of the Foundation for Shamanic Studies, defines shamanism in *The Way of the Shaman* as "a man or woman who enters an altered state of consciousness—at will—to contact and utilize an ordinarily hidden reality in order to acquire knowledge, power, and to help other persons. The shaman has at least one, and usually more, 'spirits' in his personal service" (Harner, *Way of the Shaman* 20). In the article "Science, Spirits, and Core Shamanism," from the online journal *Shamanism,* Harner also outlines two basic concepts that pervade shamanism worldwide: "Humans are part of the totality of nature, related to all other biological forms, and not superior to them" (Harner, "Science, Spirits" par. 1). He adds, "There are two realities and that the perception of each depends upon one's state of consciousness" (Harner, "Science, Spirits" par. 2). From a 1996 interview in the journal *Alternative Therapies*, "Shamanic Healing: We Are Not Alone," (reproduced in the online journal *Shamanism)*, Harner said, that from his perspective, "the practice of shamanism is a method, not a religion. It coexists with established religions in many cultures" (Horrigan and Harner, "Shamanic Healing" par. 4).

In most cases, the shaman has a specific role within his or her culture. The shaman commonly fulfills the role of counselor, prophet, priest and physician. The healing role is the one most commonly practiced by the people we will discuss in the context of their South Carolina, Pennsylvania and Virginia communities.

Most shamans or healers have received some sort of unique calling to their role as healer or other form of magical practitioner. This may be in the form of a physical sign present at birth, such as a caul, a membrane over the face of the child, which alerts those present that this is a special child. Sometimes a healer exhibits some extraordinary trait, such as the ability to enter trance states with ease or to see into the spirit world (often called second sight).

A person may be called to a life of healing because of an illness or accident, and once recovered; she or he realizes a special gift. Once this ability has manifested, it may be passed from generation to generation within a family, although it is usually only taught by one gender to the other. This heritage then becomes a form of legitimization for the healer. You will often hear someone say something like "my father was a healer and so was his mother before him, so it was natural that I would become one, too."

One final way that the role of healer is conveyed is through some divine or supernatural contact, such as the case of Biddy Early, the famous Irish cunning woman who, it was said, learned her craft as a young woman from contact with the faeries.

It is important to understand that the shaman does not see the concept of healing or even sickness itself in quite the same way as the modern medical professional, but though a more holistic lens. The shaman, therefore, treats the body, mind and spirit as an integrated whole.

As we will see, the traditional healers of South Carolina have been shamans in many aspects of the term and have served their ethnic enclaves and communities in ways often unavailable through conventional means. They have communicated with their patients in concepts and often in a language unique to their background. They have counseled, advised, healed, exorcised evil influences, entered trance to commune with alternate realities and fundamentally behaved like shamans in other parts of the world. In addition, like other shamans, they often lived on the social perimeters of their cultures and were often feared, as well as respected, for their gift of performing magical acts.

What Are Magical Acts and Magical Healings?

According to folklorist Wayland Hand, in *Magical Medicine: The Folkloric Component of Medicine in the Folk Belief, Custom and Ritual of the Peoples of Europe and America*, magical acts that are associated with healing, are "a somewhat neglected field of folk medicine" (2). They "may be thought of as being in the nature of attendant circumstances or states of being that promote the designed cure" (2).

The most common approach to the examination of such acts is to observe them in their proper context—in the place and time in which they occur. For example, the magical act of casting a spell or "setting a trick" (casting a spell) in the Hoodoo tradition involves selecting the time, such as midnight; the place, perhaps in a graveyard or at a crossroads; and the manner, such as burying the trick or tossing it over your shoulder and walking away without looking back.

The concept of place and time are also important to the act of magical or spiritual healing. Many traditions believe that the effectiveness of a healing is enhanced by performing the ritual in a special location and at a time ordained as sacred. We almost never hear of healings taking place in a restaurant, a toilet or a shopping mall. The sacred must be kept separate from the mundane and profane. An excellent example of this is the New Testament story of Jesus violently ejecting the moneylenders from the sacred space of the temple. One of the original objections against Jesus by the religious establishment of the time was that he performed healings at inappropriate times and places.

In Catholicism, wine is employed in the ritual of communion. The wine is believed to undergo a magical transformation via the ritual act of Communion into the actual blood of Christ. That ritual act, called transubstantiation, confers a further magical effect, as the blood of Christ is believed to have spiritual healing qualities. Many Protestants, especially those with injunctions against the consumption of alcohol, will employ fruit juice and forego the belief in transubstantiation, but the anticipated healing effect to body, mind and spirit is the same.

How Does a Magical Healing Really Work?

In all of the shamanic traditions I have examined in my research, there is s commonality in the magical healing process that takes two basic forms. At the simplest level, healing involves the focusing of the healer's life energy to the patient, or, the healer channeling Divine energy through his or her body to the patient. Both forms are considered to be of Divine origin, echoing the common rationale of "a gift from God."

Magical healing is not only the movement of this Divine energy to the patient by the healer's focused intent, but also the acceptance and integration of that energy by the patient. Therefore, placing the patient in a receptive frame of mind is the next task of the shaman, after diagnosis of the illness. Further, in shamanic healing, it is not necessary that the patient and healer be in the same place. For example, with the healing of animals, children and adults done from a distance, the patient's awareness of the healing is not required. A magical healer must be able to take his or her personal energy or divinely channeled source and, essentially, mold it into a separate, tangible substance to project it toward the patient from his or her own awareness.

I witnessed a dramatic form of this second type of healing in 2003, when visiting a family of Powwows (traditional German healers) near Philadelphia. During the preparation of the evening meal, one of the children was playing on the bench seat of the kitchen table when she slipped and fell, hitting her mouth on the edge of the table and splitting her lip badly. As expected, she screamed and cried, despite her mother's best efforts to calm her.

At that point, her father walked into the room and asked his wife, "Can I help her?" Without a word, the mother handed over the still screaming, wriggling child, who was bleeding profusely. The father cradled her in his arms and gently raised his hand approximately one foot above his daughter's face, whereupon she instantly went limp and silent, hanging in his arms like a rag doll. He then placed the first two fingers of his right hand a few inches from her still-bleeding lip and began to softly chant a Powwow healing chant in German. I positioned myself nearby and watched as, within seconds, the bleeding stopped, the wound closed and healing skin formed over the injured lip. He gently blew air into the child's face as if to revive her.

As she awoke, she looked up and smiled at him. He asked, "Are you okay, honey?" His daughter nodded, and he added, "All right, go on and play." He then turned to me and asked, "Was that all right?" as if seeking my approval.

"Of course," I replied. "It worked didn't it?"

As we will see later in our examination of Powwow, the shaman/healer will also separate and draw out a portion of his or her consciousness. The shaman will then give this a separate existence as an ideational construct (tangible thought form) and send it out to recover information or to act on his or her behalf or for the benefit of the client or patient. This conscious, but less tangible form of a living person is called an eidolon. *Webster's Dictionary* defines an eidolon as an "an unsubstantial image." This conceived mental construct can take any form desired or remain an invisible presence.

Such a construct can also be created unconsciously by someone experiencing a traumatic event. Everyday people often leave constructs throughout their lives, which can be sensed by children, animals, those trained to detect them or those born with an enhanced sensitivity to such energy residues.

It is important to note that the healer does more than just send energy to a patient to correct a physical or mental ailment. The shamanic healer also strives to restore a sense of psychological balance to the patient's life. This sense of balance is viewed as essential to maintaining the physical, mental and spiritual health of the person. A lack of this life-energy balance is often described as the root cause of disease in the shamanic worldview.

As illustrated above by the healing of the child's lip, the physical manifestation of the healing observed and experienced by the patient or others present may take the form of gestures, such as the healer's hand sweeping over the person's body, or the actual touch of the healer accompanied by some verbal sounds or chants. Shamans believe in the great healing power of sound, touch and breath, as transmissions of Divine energy. For example, in Powwow, chants are most commonly employed, as it is believed that energy is passed from healer to patient via the voice. There are several types of charms that have survived, which I have encountered over the years (see Appendix). Many of the spoken charms I encountered come from the popular Powwow spell-book by John George Hohman entitled *The Long Lost Friend; A Collection of Mysterious and Invaluable Arts and Remedies for Man as well as Animals*, which was first published in 1820 in Pennsylvania.

Many believe the magical healing actually takes place because of a momentary spiritual union with the Divine. The shaman enters a transcendent state of awareness, which she or he has personally cultivated as a spiritual practice.

This altered state of awareness is difficult to describe or analyze and is considered outside the realm of ordinary experience. It does not behave in an absolutely consistent manner and hence does not lend itself easily to scientific analysis or intellectual discourse.

This Divine connection cannot be forced by the intellect but must occur automatically though the chants, gestures and rituals employed to facilitate it. This is why many of the chants and gestures may not seem to have a rational basis for being performed or a direct correlation to the illness. They are subtle cues for the shaman's inner awareness. They allow the shaman to become receptive, letting the healing manifest through his or her words and actions. Healing in popular literature is often associated with the heart or emotional part of our being. During this state of heightened awareness, the shaman is not cognitively analyzing or making judgments but acting from a deeper level of consciousness where the energy can flow without interference.

Shamanic Definition of Illness

Disease and health in the shamanic worldview are seen as two sides of the same coin, not polar opposites. From this viewpoint, illness is composed of four basic causes: mental/physical, spiritual or by magical intrusion which is defined as a projected form of concentrated energy either projected by an adept toward another person or the conscious or unconscious encounter with an entity.

In the Powwow tradition, life is considered to exist as a manifestation of many levels of vibrating energy. Each level of that energy is considered another manifestation of personal reality and is often referred to as another body.

For example, what is called the astral body is considered our form in the spiritual dimension of life. We had this astral body as our primary form before birth and will have it again after death as our primary spirit form. This astral body is necessary to animate our corporeal body while we inhabit a physical form.

These layers of energy or bodies constitute the whole person, even though most of us are not fully aware of these separate presences, mistaking them for our mind and constituted personality. The Hindus refer to this illusion of our mind or constituted personality as *maya*. Following this idea of interrelated layers or dimensions of the self, if one layer is out of sync, the rest are affected, and illness or injury results. It is the healer's goal to restore that balance. Shamanic tradition may include personal counseling, as it often compliments the healing process.

Seeing the self through a shamanic perception, the various levels of our existence vibrate and fluctuate throughout our lives. These ongoing changes indicate the periods of illness and health, both physical and mental. Often the physical affects the mental, and vice versa, in what appears seamless to the individual's ordinary state of awareness.

During the diagnostic phase of the healing process, the healer questions and examines the patient for signs of imbalance. In the Powwow tradition, this is often done by passing the healer's hands over the patient to feel or sense the presence of imbalance or magical intrusion. It is important to note that physical contact does not need to take place for a diagnosis to be successful. In the first pass, the healer tries to get a sense of the person's normal energy flow. In the second, the healer is searching for an irregularity in that flow. Often, the healer's eyes are closed and he or she is in a heightened state of awareness. An imbalance is reported to feel like "darkness," or a cold or hot spot. Either way, something is out of balance or should not be there at all.

Perceiving and experiencing this energy imbalance requires a form of empathetic extension of the healer's consciousness with that of the patient, allowing the healer to enter the thoughts and feelings of the patient or victim. If the illness is caused by magical intrusion, the healer will often get a mental image of the source, whether a person, a separate entity or a projected thought form.

In healing a mental or physical imbalance, the healer must be alert to the possibility that as a result of this empathetic connection, he or she may become momentarily subject to the illness or intrusion. Because of this risk, the healer must be careful to be able to protect and disentangle his or her own consciousness from the intrusion without harm.

This ability to empathically merge with a patient takes considerable practice. There are some healers who will actually take on the illness or intrusion themselves in order to assist the person in overcoming or expelling it. This empathetic immersion is a considered a dangerous method and should only be employed in the most dire circumstances where no other options are available. It is believed that subtle forms of the negative energy can stick to the healer as a harmful residue. Regardless of the technique employed, the healer must take care to cleanse or otherwise restore his or her own physical, mental and psychic equipoise after conducting a healing or other magical act. Some healers wash with water, some clear all energies by burning such cleansing herbs as sage and some use prayer and meditation. This act of personal self-preservation is especially important where magical intrusion is determined to be the cause of the problem

Magically-Based Intrusions

A magical intrusion is considered, for our purposes, to be a method of causing physical illness, mental instability or even death to someone, usually through the focused ill-will of another person or a person who has been employed to perform this type of psychic attack or the intrusion of an outside entity into a person's sphere of existence.

The intrusion is accomplished through focusing the negative mental energy on an object in an act of sympathetic magic, which is then transferred to the victim. The methods of transference include drilling a hole in a tree, placing an item belonging to or associated with the person into the hole, then sealing it up. As the tree withers and dies, so does the intended victim.

Another method involves the placement of a physically charged object in the presence or path of the victim, resulting in a magical infection of the person. Thirdly, magical intrusion can be effected by focusing one's negative mental energy toward the intended victim. In other cultures, this is called the "evil eye." In the South Carolina Low Country, such harmful intent is called a "root." We will examine several more examples of magical intrusion in later chapters.

Should the shamanic healer detect the presence of magical intrusion, the shaman's job changes. The personal or divinely channeled energy is focused on the expulsion of the intrusive energy.

First, the source is identified and then it is countered by a variety of methods. In Powwow, it is called a "take-in-off" and in root-doctoring, "killing the root." This curse or hex removal can be as simple as praying over the victim or as complex as a series of specific rituals and cleansings. Ideally, the healer will accompany the victim back home, or to where the victim first encountered the magical intrusion. The healer will cleanse that space and install magical protective devices.

In other cases, the healer might simply prescribe, a series of activities to ensure that the intrusion will not occur again. The healer can prevent further attacks by use of a counterattack on the source of the intrusion. This form of magical practice may also include the exorcism and expulsion of a spirit entity affecting the person or space, such as during a haunting. A haunting, however, may not be necessarily negative but simply the presence of a benign entity that has chosen to occupy the same physical space as a living person.

For example, I was recently called to an elegant, upscale apartment in downtown Nashville by some friends from our church to examine and possibly expel a presence within their home. They had recently become aware of this presence, and it was causing them concern. I went with my wife and asked another gifted psychic to assist me. Upon arriving and locating the entity, we determined that it was the spirit of a young teenager, who had died many years ago, and whose spirit had moved into the attic closet. It was aware of the couple; it meant them no ill-will and simply wanted to be left alone. When we reported our findings to our friends, they decided they could live peaceably with the spirit and no expulsion was necessary.

As we can see from our examination of magical intrusion, healing has taken on an expanded role and focus to include the patient and his or her environment. This expanding role reflects the holistic view of life and its environs as intimately interrelated and interconnected.

A Healer's Mystical Life

The healer, to be effective must learn to avoid the entrapments of egotism and the illusion of personal power. She or he must learn to cultivate the Divine connection and the experience of enhanced awareness to the point that it becomes a way of life. Most healers who succeed over the long term find the need to secure the guidance of a mentor or a spirit guide who can teach them and direct their growth.

The learning process is akin to one of spiritual growth and can be fraught with problems, as the healer begins to uncover his or her own layers of personal existence. Many times, the dark and hidden parts of ourselves emerge as we open ourselves to the Divine, often causing tears, terror and many "dark nights of the soul."

Many novice shamans find this process too unsettling or disturbing, especially when they encounter the world of spirits and other experiences outside their normal realms of perception. These sincere people may still adopt a lower level of practice, such as only healing superficial wounds: cuts, bruises and burns, becoming a "charmer" as in the British traditions, which we will discuss in more detail in the chapter on the Appalachian Granny tradition.

One person I interviewed said that, as his consciousness expanded, he became terrified that "there would be nothing left of me." However, should the shaman grow past that fear and persist in this inner journey, different layers of his or her consciousness will emerge and an entirely new view of reality will present itself to his expanding consciousness.

The final, direct experience of the Divine is a form of emergence from the cocoon of mundane existence into a new world of expanded awareness. One person described it as a feeling of joy and love beyond the realm of romantic love and desire, but an incredible feeling of wholeness and completeness. As a result, the shaman's conventional experience of religion and faith take on a new and expanded form.

"I knew in that moment that Jesus was real!" one woman from Kentucky exclaimed. "More real than even me. . . . I still go to church, but a lot of what goes on just doesn't mean anything anymore. I'm just sitting there feeling God everywhere and knowing I can't tell a soul or they would think I was crazy," she concluded. This woman had learned the wisdom of keeping her expanded awareness to herself. It is no wonder that most religious organizations do not traditionally support this form of spiritual practice, as it tends to eliminate the need for a clerical mediator or dependence on group approval.

The Necessity of Solitude

This expanded awareness often compels the shaman to retreat from the conventional world at time, whether by choosing to live away from urban areas or by creating sacred, protected space as a personal sanctuary. This retreat should not be misinterpreted as a rejection of society or everyday life, but as a natural result of expanded sensory awareness.

It has often been noted by those that hike for long periods in the wilderness that, as they return to their usual environment, they experience the auditory noise level as a loud roaring that is unpleasant, until the adjustment to the modern world has been made. Similarly, the shaman often has to retreat from the world and all its distractions, until he or she can re-establish contact with the mundane.

The path of the shaman or mystic is not without personal perils and costs. Our modern society is not ready or socially configured to accommodate the presence or actions of the shaman. Those wishing to sincerely pursue this spiritual path must accept that, for most of their remaining time in this life, they will walk alone on life's path and cultivate social invisibility. This is clearly not a path for those who need the affirmation of others or who need to share their spiritual lives with others.

Such solitude and increased awareness is more easily found in non-urban areas where nature's ongoing processes provide a way of renewing and staying connected to the Divine. This desire for Divine connection can become a consuming passion, a hunger that must be nurtured, for a shaman to remain personally balanced and to perform the tasks required.

To be practical, however, the modern shaman must learn to manage the Divine experience and still reconnect with everyday awareness to remain a functioning member of our society. The rent must be paid, food acquired and other social obligations met. Some Asian cultures adopt and care for the hermit, shaman or mystic. Our Western society, regrettably, usually sees only an unstable, non-functional person who needs psychiatric help because he or she is out of sync with the concepts of scientific rationalism in the greater society.

It will be clear to the reader from this introduction that during the past thirty years I have not remained simply a detached observer in my research into these shamanic traditions. I committed many years ago to provide, as best as I am able, spiritually-based shamanic services to those that sincerely request them. I do not charge for these services, as they are acts of my own faith in the Divine and its active presence in our lives. I tend to operate within the Powwow tradition as it is the one with which I am most comfortable.

I acknowledge that for some readers, this presentation of my exploration and immersion in the healing traditions of root doctor, Powwow and similar magical practices may seem far-fetched and hard to believe. I, too, have struggled with my own incredulity over much of what I have witnessed and participated in. During the past thirty years, I have come to see these traditional magical healings, their nurturing and practice, as a gift from the Divine. I hope those who pick up this book will remain open-minded enough to continue reading as I recall the long, sometimes strange, path that has led me to revere these ancient spiritual practices. If you find this recounting to be beyond your ability to accept, then I understand and fondly bid you farewell.

CHAPTER ONE

Beneath the Spanish Moss:
The World of the Root Doctor

History is the version of past events that people have decided to agree upon.
— Napoleon Bonaparte, (1769–1821)

The thing always happens that you really believe in; and the belief in a thing makes it happen.
— Frank Lloyd Wright, (1869–1959)

FOR MANY OF US growing up in the 1960s rural South, the world of ghosts, witches and magic was never far away. Grandparents and parents often told hair-raising stories of mysterious happenings and eerie events as a form of entertainment, as children sat entranced in wide-eyed amazement. The idea of a ghost or witch out there in the dark filled many a night with excitement and wonder. In many homes, the sense of the presence of a beloved, deceased family member was often noted with comfort and the reassurance that we would someday "meet on that golden shore."

In this era, before the Internet and television's mindless absorption of our free time, we often felt we could sense that which was unseen, and provided we didn't make too much of a fuss about it, we were free to believe in the miraculous without fear of rebuke or censure.

When we became ill, home remedies and therapies were employed first to treat many types of sickness, and prayers were an integral part of the healing process. Doctors were expensive and were consulted only when traditional healing methods were not effective.

Sometimes, parents adhered more to modern ideas and dismissed the old traditional remedies—both herbal and spiritual—as superstition. As is not uncommon in close-knit, extended families, children often had a special rapport and respect for their grandparents. We learned not to be too quick in dismissing traditional beliefs or to ignore things seen just out of the range of normal sight. Perhaps as a result of this close connection with the older generation, as children, we were more open to the miraculous and spiritual in nature, although such sensitivities also seemed to run in certain families.

For example, I can remember as a teenager watching a friend's mother scrying into a large brass bowl to gain knowledge of geographically distant events. We were always respectful of our elders, no matter how eccentric, and we would assume there were many things in this world beyond our understanding. For us, this other spiritual world existed in addition to and often as a compliment to a clearly defined tradition of attending church on Sunday. One was the public expression of faith and the other a more private one. As a result, old beliefs were internalized and retained as an intimate part of our personalities.

A Child's Personal Look Back: Society and Race in the Rural South

Contrary to the popular picture painted by the national media of white and black race relations in the South during the late 1950s and 1960s, in many areas, while living separate public lives, many blacks and whites privately regarded each other with acceptance and respect.

Children of both races were taught to respect adults, regardless of their color. I cannot imagine what would have happened to me had my folks discovered I had participated in some sort of racially motivated incident. Such things were "just not done by decent Christian people," as my mother would say. Racism, while socially tolerated, was also considered by many whites an offense against the God that made us all. This sort of racism was a Catch-22 situation, and actually repressive to everyone involved in the culture. Few Southern whites felt they could risk challenging the prevailing social mores, so there developed an odd paradigm of public and private socially mixed messages.

At the time, many churches would refuse to seat an African American during a service, yet the children's Sunday school would be singing "Jesus Loves the Little Children" with the words "Red, and yellow, black and white, they are precious in his sight, Jesus loves the little children of the world."

This odd, disjointed social paradigm was also a part of our everyday lives.

In reality, in the 1950s and 1960s and even today, the private under-current and public expression of racism probably has as much to do with social positioning as actual race. Someone had to occupy the bottom rung of society, given the similar histories of exploitation and manipulation of the poor whites and African Americans in the South. The dominant socio-economic class had long understood that they could control both groups by effectively pitting one against the other along racial lines. It worked effectively during Reconstruction and it still functions today with the same sad results for both groups.

I would never attempt to paint a sentimental or beneficent picture of the social situation that existed in the 1960s South. On a personal level, however, it was during those times that some barriers began to crumble.

Here is an example from my own childhood. My mother, who was a career woman in a managerial position in the 1950s, which was unusual for that time and place, fell ill. Her condition required surgery, and during her recovery, she hired an African American woman to help her with the housekeeping. In those days, it was the custom that the paid help would take their meals and breaks on the back porch, and not with the family. My mother, however, thought otherwise. "If she is good enough to work in my home, she's good enough to sit and eat with us at my table!" she replied, as some neighbors raised objections to the violation of this established social protocol.

After this incident, my mother was shunned by those neighbors. Yet, more than forty years later, she and her African American housekeeper have maintained their friendship and still visit and talk to this day.

Was this situation atypical? I do not know, but I suspect that for every act of bigotry and intolerance during that time, there was possibly a private one of kindness and respect. I also suspect that these expressions were more common among women than men.

Women, both black and white, shared the common bond of gender-based restrictions, which carried the real impact of economic and social repression. The difference was in the degree to which it was expressed. I am not making excuses for the terrible system of racial segregation that debased and confined both cultures. It was a cultural system that desperately needed to

change then and must continue to evolve. I am not attempting to excuse
or fully explain this complex situation. I am offering a bit of personal perspective, based on my own observations as a boy growing up in Columbia,
South Carolina, during this period.

One must also remember that unlike the ghettos of the urban north,
many blacks and whites in the South often lived in close physical proximity to each other. In the early 1960s, as segregation was lifted in the
public schools, as often as not, the social barriers propagated by adult fears,
ingrained bigotry and simple ignorance broke down within the innocence
of childhood. Friendships developed out of the wonderful activity of play.
It was often through this play that the white kids learned the stories and
lore around the legendary figures known as the root doctor or conjure man
or conjure woman.

First Glimpses of the Root Doctor or Hoodoo Culture

In 1965, my family moved to a suburb near Irmo, South Carolina, which
was fifteen miles northwest of the capitol city of Columbia. At that time,
the area was still distinctly rural. It was there that I first heard the word
"root doctor." As boys engaged in our endless games we would often here
someone exclaim "I'm going to put the root on you!" or "I'm going to
see the root doctor and he'll fix you!" These idle taunts belayed a powerful
social presence that few of us understood. We suspected there was a reality
that existed behind the everyday one of school, church and play. We heard
stories of these powerful beings who could curse and heal, transverse the
worlds of the living and the dead and were to be afforded the greatest
respect and deference.

Historically, the traditions of the conjure man, conjure woman or root
doctor came over with the Africans as they were brought to colonial America
as slaves. Among these Africans were their tribal healers or shamans. The
names that subsequently developed for their shamanic practice included root
working, conjure, witch doctoring, tricking and Hoodoo.

Modern occult authority Catherine Yronwode defines the commonly
used term "Hoodoo" on the extensive Lucky Mojo website. In the section
called "Hoodoo in Theory and Practice," she writes in the article "Hoodoo:

African American Magic," that Hoodoo is "an American term, originating in the nineteenth century or earlier for African American folk magic" (Yronwode 1). Yronwode continues,

> Hoodoo consists of a large body of African folkloric practices and beliefs with a considerable admixture of American Indian botanical knowledge and European folklore. Although most of its adherents are black, contrary to popular opinion, it has always been practiced by both whites and blacks in America. ("Magic" 1)

She goes on to describe the variations applied to the word Hoodoo:

> Hoodoo is used as a noun to name both the system of magic ("He used hoodoo on her") and its practitioners ("Doctor Buzzard was a great hoodoo in his day"). In the 1930s, some practitioners used the noun "hoodooism" (analogous with "occultism") to describe their work, but that term has dropped out of common parlance. Hoodoo is also an adjective ("he layed a hoodoo trick for her") and a verb ("she hoodooed that man until he couldn't love no one but her"). (Yronwode, "Magic" par. 2)

The word Hoodoo permeated the language and culture of the rural South; it has appeared in the lyrics of hundreds of traditional blues and folk songs dating back to the early 19th century.

As to the source of the term "root"—as in a charm or a person known as a root doctor—it is also rooted in history with multiple definitions. Strictly speaking, the actual term "root" refers to a man-made object created by the root doctor that contains herbs, symbols and other objects needed to affect the spell. The roots I have seen in my own fieldwork have been in bottles, sewn in packets of cloth or tied together in a bundle Most have been "charged" with something to activate them. In her book, *Black Magic: Religion and the African American Conjuring Tradition,* historian Yvonne Chireau says, "Root work characterized the style of utilizing certain natural objects in the performance of ritual" (277). In the chapter "Doctors and Root Doctors: Patients Who Use Both," from *Herbal and Magical Medicine: Traditional Healing Today,* Holly Matthews says root in regard to this magical system is "because plant roots are an important component of magical spells that are used to cause illnesses and of the remedies used to cure them" (69). In many parts of the Carolinas and Georgia, the terms Hoodoo and root work are used interchangeably, as they are in this book.

The Seeds of Hoodoo Culture

Faith Mitchell cites three factors leading to the development of the distinct African American culture found in the Low Country of South Carolina and Georgia, in her book *Hoodoo Medicine: Gullah Herbal Remedies*. These three factors are the large proportion of black slaves imported to South Carolina, the geographic and social isolation in which the slaves often found themselves after the end of the Civil War, and laws that allowed for the direct importation of slaves from the African subcontinent to that coastal region commonly known as the Low Country.

As Robert Olwell notes in *Masters, Slaves and Subjects: The Culture of Power in the South Carolina Low Country, 1740-1790*, the term Low Country is generally used to refer to an area that "extends along South Carolina's Atlantic shore for approximately two hundred miles and inland for fifty miles or so" (10).

South Carolina was originally settled from existing British colonies in Barbados. The Low Country did not provide the new settlers with a land like home or the Caribbean. The settlers found wide coastal plains, swamps infested with snakes and mosquitoes, and hurricanes that would sweep in without warning and devastate everything in their path. This was not an easy place to secure politically or in which to prosper without a significant labor pool. The importation of slaves directly from Africa and the Caribbean provided that labor, and in doing so, forever changed the culture and history of the colony.

A relatively unknown aspect of this period was that in the early days of the colonies, many de facto slaves were gleaned from the poorer classes of the British Isles, which was already an also common practice in the British colonies of the Caribbean. The terms often used for this forced importation of human beings was called transportation and indentured servitude, which to the casual reader sounds like a form of labor exchange for the payment of passage to the colonies or a just sentence for some moral infraction. In the *Dictionary of Afro-American Slavery*, Robert McColley notes, "Englishmen, in the early seventeenth century, used the word *servant* when they meant *slave* in our sense, and, indeed, white Southerners invariably used *servant* until 1865 and beyond" (781).

The modern American must remember that the aristocratic citizens of the American colonies carried with them the perceptions and prejudices of English society towards those in poverty, non-Christians, foreigners and non-Caucasians. Personal wealth and social success was seen as resulting from Divine favor and hence, those without it deserved their wretched fate and more.

According to Stephen Talty's 2000 article "Spooked: The White Slave Narratives," published in *Transition,* this was not a period of great compassion for the suffering of others. Most citizens at least partially agreed with Virginia Tidewater planter and philosopher of slavery, George Fitzhugh, when he said, "Some are born with saddles on their backs and the riding does them good" (Talty 69-70). This rationalization led the wealthy planters to believe the poor were actually uplifted by their servitude. This attitude toward the lower classes survived well into the 20th century. I can clearly remember during the period of the Civil Rights movement hearing unselfconscious comments like "but we were good to our Negroes, we looked after them, they're like children, you know" and "Poor things, nothing but white trash. They just can't help themselves."

In many cases, the poor of the British Isles often sold themselves to a sea captain or company to avoid debtor's prison. Working class people could be arrested and classified as criminals for an incredibly wide variety of petty offenses, including not attending church, being unemployed, not being able to pay their debts, being a member of the losing side in a rebellion or a political rival to the government. Many were also kidnapped, including thousands of children, and shipped to the colonies under horrific conditions where, if they survived, they were sold into a life of frequent brutality and hard labor until they ran away or died. This indenturing, transportation and eventual sale of thousands of individuals and, in many cases, their entire families, became an economically lucrative business that thrived throughout the colonial period. The wealthy planter society that personally despised and exploited these people had financially supported this system until it became clear, as with the Caribbean slave experience, that enslaved whites proved physically unsuited for the semi-tropical climate of the Low Country and easily succumbed to disease and hardship. Native Americans likewise proved difficult to manage and, like their white counterparts, could slip away and blend into the social fabric of the colony. The African slave was physically suited to the environment and could be more easily identified should he or she try to escape. Later in the colonial period, after two violent social backlashes by the poor class of whites against their treatment by the landed aristocracy, the planter society conceded some social status to the poor white in return for social and racial loyalty. According to Olwell, it is considered by some that they

> . . . were often suspected of having too much familiarity with the slaves, they also filled the ranks of the town watch, the parish slave patrol and found employment as overseers on the large estates. (45)

Many also became tenant farmers and most never realized the promise of true freedom and opportunity of the new world.

The Impact of the Africans

According to the 2004 PBS television series, "Africans in America: The Terrible Transformation, Part 1: 1450–1750," in the early days of the colonies:

> Many Africans and poor whites—most of the laborers came from the English working class—stood on the same ground. Black and white women worked side-by-side in the fields. Black and white men who broke their servant contract were equally punished. ("Indentured" 1)
>
> All were indentured servants. During their time as servants, they were fed and housed. Afterwards, they would be given what were known as "freedom dues," which usually included a piece of land and supplies, including a gun. Black-skinned or white-skinned, they became free. ("Identured" 1)

An insidious, racist ideology began to develop that was applied specifically to the African Americans, while a similar, but class-oriented ideology developed toward the poor whites. Both groups were seen as social inferiors and therefore deserving of scorn and exploitation. The particular racial ideology applied to African Americans sought to secure and insure social dominance based on ideas of inherent biological and mental inferiority and often characterized both slaves and former slaves as less than completely human. Even religious texts were employed as a rationalization for the continued subjugation and mistreatment of an entire race of people. Social groups who wish to dominate a race, ethnic group or gender throughout history, have used religion and later pseudo-science to justify their cruelty and maintain their social status. As far back as the Old Testament, we find many written accounts of those societies whom the Israelites conquered demonized as corrupt, evil and deserving of conquest and destruction. Some elements of human behavior seem constant throughout the ages.

Historian David Blight says in "Africans in America":

> . . . [the] disorder that the indentured servant system had created made racial slavery to southern slaveholders much more attractive, because what were black slaves now? Well, they were a permanent dependent labor force, which could be defined as a people set apart. They were racially set apart. They were outsiders. They were strangers and in many ways throughout the world, slavery has taken root, especially where people are considered outsiders and can be put in a permanent status of slavery. ("Indentured" 3)

The impact of the presence of African American culture on life in the South Carolina and Georgia Low Country is impossible to understate. In the online article "Understanding Slavery: The Lives of Eighteenth Century African-Americans," found on the South Carolina Information Highway website, published by the Chicora Foundation, it is noted that

> . . . the history of South Carolina is inexorably intertwined with slavery. Everything on the plantation—the roads, the buildings, the fences, the gardens and the crops—was the result of African American sweat and blood. There likely would be no South Carolina history were it not for the labors of the African Americans brought to these shores in slave ships. (1)

The predominant crops grown in the developing plantation system in coastal South Carolina were rice, indigo and livestock, which required experience and specialized skills. Faith Mitchell points out that many slaves "may have had prior experience tending herds" (16) and were familiar with the cultivation of rice in Africa, making these particular people very valuable

to the growing agricultural environment. Most of the slaves imported to
the South Carolina coast and Georgia through the ports of Charleston and
Savannah were from the west coast of Africa from countries now known as
Gambia, Ghana and Nigeria.

Culture by Sheer Force of Numbers

The importance the role of the slave population in South Carolina's cultural
history is hard to underestimate, according to "The Lives of African-American Slaves in Carolina During the 18th Century":

> South Carolina had a clear black majority from about 1708 through most
> of the eighteenth century. By 1720 there were about 18,000 people living
> in South Carolina and 65% of these were enslaved African Americans. In
> St. James Goose Creek, a parish just north of Charles Towne, there were
> only 535 whites and 2,027 black slaves. (1)

This numerical imbalance in population led to a near constant fear of
slave revolts among whites and a brutally repressive society for the slave.
Curiously, this fear also brought an odd blending of African and Anglo
cultures while maintaining a severe imbalance of social and political power.
As Frank Tannenbaum noted in *Slave and Citizen: The Negro in the Americas*,
"Nothing escaped the influence of slaves and slavery, nothing and no one"
(117). Various patterns of speech and habits, such as cooking and attitudes,
were exchanged between whites and blacks, yet they lived socially worlds
apart with many different gradations and strata within their societies. There
were also many people in a sort of social limbo due to their mixed racial
heritage that was, while officially frowned upon, quietly tolerated.

Many slaves initially resisted attempts to Christianize them and in the
Southeast, there existed no legal or cultural desire by the white population
to do so. Carolyn Morrow Long reminds us in *Spiritual Merchants: Religion,
Magic and Commerce*, that "English Common Law, unlike the Black Codes
of the Catholic Slave trading countries of France, Spain, and Portugal, did
not acknowledge the rights of slaves as human beings; they were viewed
strictly as property" (72).

Several authors have indicated that slaveholders feared that the slave's
conversion to was viewed with suspicion as a possible step toward some

level of equality and legal status. Long indicates that only after several slave revolts during the colonial period were the slave owners finally "persuaded that Christianization would make the slaves more docile" (73).

It was within this cultural and social confusion that traditional African practices were adapted to their new environment and, in turn, inserted themselves into the new plantation slave culture. This process preserved elements of the African heritage while becoming a cultural hybrid. It was this largely invisible cultural system that included Hoodoo.

Hoodoo as a Cultural System Distinct from Voodoo

In her exploration of the hoodoo tradition, Catherine Yronwode defines this magical system as one different from the Voodoo-based slave society of New Orleans and the Gulf Coast. In the section "What Hoodoo Is," on the webpage "Hoodoo: African American Magic," Yronwode says Hoodoo:

> . . . places emphasis on personal magical power and thus it lacks strong links to any specific form of theology and can be adapted to any one of several forms of outward religious worship. Although an individual practitioner may take on students, Hoodoo is structured along an obvious hierarchical system. Teachings and rituals are handed down from a one practitioner to another, but there are no priests or priestesses and no division between initiates and laity (par. 2)

Another aspect of this cultural hybrid is the difference between the magical medical practices of the slave culture of South Carolina and Georgia and the one that developed in New Orleans.

The Voodoo culture of New Orleans survives today beyond the garish shows produced for the tourist. Voodoo rituals blend at least two distinct religions and cultures: African native religions and Roman Catholicism, as practiced in the delta region of Louisiana. Voodoo practices invoke many gods and goddesses from African native religions, as well as calling on the power of Catholic saints in its magical practices.

The Hoodoo practice of root doctoring or conjure employs no specific gods or goddesses. This may be due to the predominance of Protestant-based Christianity in the Carolinas and Georgia, which teaches, according to James Kirkland in *Herbal and Magical Medicine: Traditional Healing Today*, that

> . . . the individual lives in a hostile world where the forces of God are

pitted against the forces of the devil in a daily struggle for control. Illness and misfortune are likely to result whenever the individual fails to maintain a balance between these competing forces, whether natural or magical. (71–72)

Hoodoo and Root doctoring as a system does acknowledge the presence of spirits and a spirit world, but it is more akin to the traditional African belief in animism.

It must be stated at this point that root doctoring or Hoodoo is also a distinct tradition from Haitian Voudou and Santeria in the same way it differs from New Orleans Voodoo: the syncretic blend of traditions varies within each practice, based on culture, language, customs, and evolved religious practices. Hoodoo did, however, adopt ideas and practices from other cultures, including Esoteric German Christianity and the Jewish mystical tradition of Kabbalah. This adoption occurred as a result of commerce when magical treatises like "The Black Pullet," "The Sixth and Seventh Books of Moses," and the so-called "spurious" magical writings of Albertus Magnus were typically offered through the catalogs of Jewish-owned curio companies like King Novelty and Clover Horn, according to Yronwode ("Admixtures" 11). For example, Low Country root doctors began to use psalms from the Christian Bible as chants and incantations from a book called *Secrets of the Psalms*, a cheaply made paperback of dubious authorship and origin based very loosely on the use of the psalms in the Kabbalah.

There have been quite a few inexpensively produced compilations of spells sold by such curio shops as mentioned above. As many of the spells, formulas and ritual practices contained in these titles were adopted and contributed to the development of root and Hoodoo practices, a mention of a few historic titles is appropriate to the discussion of resources available to the interested or would-be practitioner.

Several of these small magical texts have circulated for more than a century in Powwow and Hoodoo circles as spell-books. John George Hohman's *The Long Lost Friend, The Sixth and Seventh Books of Moses,* and *Albertus Magnus* are the most well known. They provided recipes for potions and plasters, along with spells for all manner of purposes from colic in horses, spellbinding thieves, curing snakebite and banishment of evil spirits. Many of these books were compilations of charms and spells from many, often questionable, sources but as they met a need, they were widely accepted and distributed.

In 1974, I found a mail order reprint copy of Hohman's *Powwows; or The Long Lost Friend: A Collection of Mysterious and Invaluable Arts and Remedies for Man as Well as Animals.* Several years ago, I bought another copy from Amazon.com as my older one was falling apart. Hohman, at least, was an early compiler of the folk remedies he knew from his native land and from his new-found home. According to what is known of him, Hohman traveled extensively in the early 19th century German and Swiss communities peddling his book of remedies with modest success. After his death, *The Long Lost Friend* was reproduced throughout the 19th century by small local presses in limited production runs. In this century, it has been sold as a cheap reprint by so-called novelty houses, whose merchandise also included lotions, potions, charms, religious talismans, etc., for the rural and newly urbanized Appalachian, German and African American communities. This is a remarkable publishing record for a rather unremarkable booklet. It stands as testament to the enduring quality of the private culture of family traditions.

Although we have seen some similarities in books and materials used in various traditions, the ritual differences are significant. Another difference between the Hoodoo and Voodoo traditions is found in their respective ritual behaviors. In New Orleans Voodoo, rituals were often semi-public events involving numerous people with specific tasks to perform in order for the event to be successful. In many cases, drums, dancing and chants were employed around a permanent or semi-permanent altar. The rituals were led by a group of special dedicants or a single priest or priestess. As the worship service progressed, members of the ritual team would enter trance and become possessed by the Gods or spirits summoned for the ritual. In this state of trance, they would convey blessings, information or simply adopt and emulate the known behaviors of the Gods.

In Hoodoo, formal group rituals of any sort were a rare exception. Most root doctors understood that the group rituals were being performed in and by the local Christian church. The magical, ritual practices therefore were often conducted in private by one individual or with one assistant. The act of formal religious worship simply was not a part of the practice.

The Golden Age of the Root Doctor

After the Civil War, much of the land that comprised the old plantations and many small farms existed for decades in a state of cultural isolation. These small, isolated areas suffered from a form of state and local governmental indifference and neglect that lasted well into the 20th century. Many African Americans in the Low Country or on the coastal islands lived without significant contact with the greater American culture or even regional societies. Faith Mitchell, in *Hoodoo Medicine*, says, "... in the 1930s, the first bridges connecting the Sea Islands to the mainland were built" (17). This isolation factor was especially true for the Gullah culture of the Sea Islands, just off the coast near Beaufort and Savannah. Gullah culture was essentially ignored by the white world after the Civil War; hence, it grew and retained many elements of its African roots in its dialect, music, spirituality, arts and customs. During the 1920s, according to leading anthropologist Melville Herskowits, in William Pollitzer's *The Gullah People and their African Heritage,* the Gullah culture was "very African" (12). In such social isolation, many of these people reached into their collective memory and sought guidance through their heritage. Out of that heritage emerged people who became adept in healing, interpreting the environment and dealing with the unknown—as they perceived it—which included the belief in the world of spirits and magic.

During the period of slavery, each plantation or community had a shaman who addressed these spiritual issues and provided the necessary magical services. These individuals, like their African counterparts, were often chosen and groomed from childhood for their roles. Pollitzer emphasizes that this grooming and training of the shaman is a direct transmission of traditional African spiritual concepts and says, "no sharp line can be drawn between religion, magic and healing, especially in Africa and the Sea Islands" (143). Before the war, slaves sought help from the root doctor for illness, spiritual guidance and even protection from the pain of their servitude. This was done in secret for fear of reprisal from the slave owner. In his 1849 memoir, *Narrative of the Life and Adventures of Henry Bibb, an American Slave,* the author recanted several instances of seeking and securing magical assistance from a root doctor to avoid being ill-treated by his master/owner. As with their African counterparts, the root doctors were respected and often feared because of their ability to summon and handle unknown forces. These magical professionals adopted and adapted local herbs and the magical practices of other cultures, such as the Scots-Irish whites and Native Americans, to create a powerful syncretism of beliefs and practices. One such practice was the use of a bottle to trap and contain an evil spirit and as a method of casting a spell. F. Roy Johnson, in his book *The Fabled Doctor Jim Jordon: A Story of Conjure,* indicates that although the root doctor existed before the Civil War, these practitioners only made a prominent impact on Southern society and culture after the war. During Reconstruction, former slaves were without adequate health or spiritual support systems. The root doctor had magical practice and knowledge of herbal lore to restore the health and well-being of those whom suffered from the three recognized types of illness: natural, spiritual and unnatural. No longer suppressed by the slave owners, root doctors found a fertile ground for their magical systems.

Three recognized types of illnesses

1. **Natural:** The practice of Hoodoo developed a classification of illness into those of natural, spiritual and unnatural forces. Add to this idea the traditional of the African view that health and happiness result from a balance of the body, mind and spirit. This holistic view of health led to the idea that illness resulting from natural causes came from "a violation of the balance or harmony believed present in the physical world" (Kirkland 72). Therefore, a person's physical, mental and spiritual health could be healed by restoring this natural balance of all three elements. In my fieldwork, I discovered that many of my informants made use of both conventional physicians and root doctors, without any sense of conflict or confusion. Each health care provider has a specified role in the maintenance of good health. The most common treatment by root doctors for natural illness was the preparation of an herbal remedy. Most root doctors were master herbalists who were trained by their mentors or members of the community. The knowledge and use of herbs was widespread in the Low Country. According to Yronwode, in *Hoodoo Herb and Root Magic: A Materia Magica of African-American Conjure and Traditional Formulary, Giving the Spiritual Uses of Natural Herbs, Roots, Minerals, and Zoological Curios,* another

source for this knowledge was contained in a 16th-century belief in the "Doctrine of Signatures," from Genesis 1:29, which is the idea that "every plant was put on this Earth by God for the use of mankind" (18).

According to the Doctrine of Signatures, one could locate and identify the use of an herb by a particular physical characteristic of the plant, which resembled the organ or part of the body it was Divinely assigned to cure. For example, a heart-shaped flower or leaf could be an indication that this herb was meant to treat illnesses of the heart.

2. **Spiritual:** In the realm of spiritual illness, it is believed that we can also become vulnerable to illness as a result of some act of moral turpitude, which will leave us more vulnerable to physical illness and spiritual or unnatural predations. A healthy mind and body was considered a Divine reward for moral fortitude and ethical adherence to conventional moral precepts. Many times in my childhood and especially during my adolescence, I can remember illnesses and being asked by my family what I could have done to bring these maladies upon myself. In *Herbal and Magical Medicine*, Holly Matthews says, "The victims of root work are often those individuals who have lost God's protection because of sins committed in the past" (79). According to Wilbur Watson in *Black Folk Medicine: The Therapeutic Significance of Faith and Trust,* illness was seen as "the result of willful violation of sacred beliefs or of sin such as adultery, theft or murder" (2). It is believed, for example, that a woman who has seduced another woman's lover or husband is particularly vulnerable to a curse from the woman she has insulted by her wrong actions. In one sense, a spiritual illness is the karmic or cause-and-effect result of the old adage, "what goes around, comes around." The effects of this kind of illness can be lessened or cured by traditional repentance and an attempt at retribution, such as returning the item stolen or a sincere apology to those who were initially wronged.

3. **Unnatural:** Unnatural illness, on the other hand, was seen as imposed upon or caused by the harmful actions of an outside force, either human or a non-physical entity. According to my informants, there is no definitive way to prepare for an unnatural illness (or magical

assault), although many people take care to provide themselves with ongoing protection in the form of a charm. They may wear the charm upon their person and or place magical protective devices in and around their home. Examples of protective charms include wearing a piece of silver jewelry. If the silver turns black over a very short period of time (even overnight), the tarnish is a clear indication of the presence of evil or that harmful forces have been directed against you. Placing a large piece of iron under your bed or a line of salt on your windowsill will provide protection to the home. One can also secure a personal protective root/charm from a qualified root doctor. This type of charm should be carried or worn for protection. Even so, I was once told by a young African American root doctor from Columbia (SC), "If I want to get to you, I will." He then added, "I'll come in the night, in your dreams, and you'll never know what hit you. Most white folks like to pretend that if they don't believe in it, they're safe, sure, just go on thinking that." For whatever bravado he may have been exhibiting at that moment, he said it with sincere conviction.

To remedy this type of illness required the services of the minister or, failing that, the conjure doctor who would usually employ a combination of therapies to rid the afflicted person of this negative influence. Often the treatment would work, and the illness would abate. If it did not, as Long points out in *Spiritual Merchants: Religion, Magic and Commerce*, "the failure was blamed on the victim for waiting too long to seek help or for not following the instructions" of the root doctor (78). The signs of an unnatural illness were many and varied from a general feeling of uneasiness, an unexplained rash, sharp pains or numbness in the extremities, a feeling of disassociation and withdrawal from the world and people, sudden emotional outburst, irrational behavior, even the feeling that something is crawling inside you. Some informants describe this last symptom as "like having snakes in your body." All my informants agreed that in such situations, time was critical and the root doctor's help must be secured as soon as possible before this curse "takes hold of you." If allowed to develop, the consequences can only be tragic.

I was introduced to an elderly African American woman known as "Granny Harmon" by a classmate, who was her grandson. Mrs. Harmon, a retired schoolteacher told me of a time during her childhood when her older sister was accused of stealing another woman's lover. Apparently, the woman scorned sought the services of a root doctor near their home in Orangeburg, South Carolina, and had a curse placed upon Mrs. Harmon's sister. Soon this sister became listless, refusing to eat and unable to sleep even after a hard day's work. She would pace her room, complaining of pains in her leg and manifesting scratches on her arms and back. She eventually became bed-ridden, lying motionless and staring at the ceiling. She was plagued with horrendous nightmares, and the entire family became concerned for her physical and mental stability. The local minister was called in, but his blessing and exorcism had little effect. Finally, in desperation, the family summoned a woman from a neighboring community known for her ability to "take off the root and kill it."

When the root doctor arrived, she examined the older sister, who was, by this time, almost comatose and unresponsive to vocal commands or to touch. After sending most of the family out into the hall, she began to search the room where the sister lay. After some time, she found a charm that looked like a carrot wrapped in cloth, which had been nailed in the dark recesses of the closet. As she held it out to show to the family, the sister shrieked and sat upright in her bed. The healer then walked out onto the front porch and plunged the root into a bucket of salt water, which she had asked the family to prepare before her visit. As she plunged the root into the salt water, the older sister shrieked again and fell back onto her bed. When the family rushed to her side, they found her responsive for the first time in days.

I learned that salt water is widely believed to be a neutralizer of negative psychic energy. When I asked what happened next, I learned that the healer/root doctor came back into the house and "laid a blessing on Sister." She also helped to psychically secure the room from future harm by placing salt in the windows and giving the sister a charm to hang on her bedpost. She then instructed the family on how to protect the entire household and what to watch for should the attacks resume.

"What happened to the root?" I asked. "Oh, she took it off with her.

I guess she got rid of it." The sister soon recovered her health and mental well-being and was never troubled again in this way. She apparently told her sister that being cursed was "like having something on your back and in your head, weighing you down and stealing your life."

A repertoire of magical skills

There is a common modern belief among those who view these phenomena from the outside that the person to be attacked must be made aware that he or she is under attack for the curse to work. No one with whom I have spoken as an informant felt that knowing about the attack was necessary, or that the educational level or cultural background of the person being attacked had any effect on the outcome. James E. McTeer, of Beaufort, South Carolina, was a root doctor and the local sheriff. McTeer once echoed my Columbia informant when he told me I was an easy target for psychic attack, precisely because I was educated and was given to trying to find a rational explanation for everything. "You are easier to get to because you don't recognize or accept what is happening to you," he said. "A person from around here will run quick to the root doctor to get it (the curse) taken off and they'll be okay. You will wander around trying to rationally figure it out until you're in a hell of a state." As we will see later in this book, an attack can come suddenly, without warning and without provocation. Therefore, in addition to healing physical illnesses with herbs and potions, a set of magical abilities became part of the repertoire of the root doctor, which includes the following skills:

The first magical skill expected of the root doctor is the ability to recognize the presence of, and then be able to remove, a curse or "trick" placed on an individual by an outside force, which then causes an unnatural illness. The root doctor may treat the person in his office or travel to the person's residence and locate the offending root that has been placed or hidden there. When found, the root doctor will ceremoniously remove the root and take it away or "kill" it on the spot. In several accounts, the root doctor, after killing the root (rendering it harmless), offered the root to the victim as a souvenir. One African American informant from Columbia described burying or burning the root as the best way of destroying its power, while another maintained that water, especially salt water, would render the root harmless. Other common charms for causing harm might be: a jar or bottle filled with sharp objects, a specific harmful herb, dirt from a graveyard or specially prepared powder like "goofer-dust" (to further enhance the negative effect), a personal item from the intended victim to personalize the charm, and possibly a medium to contain it like oil, urine or whiskey along with an empowering or animating ingredient like a lodestone.

The magical second skill expected of the root doctor is the ability to help restore the social balance created by some act of magical retribution. First, the root doctor identifies the attacking party, then helps the victim turn the tables on the tormentor, by magically acting on their behalf. This is done by turning the spell back onto the person believed to have perpetrated the magical aggression. A patient may be given a powder to spread or a charm to bury to reverse the curse or to inflict revenge on their enemy.

I had a young female informant (whom I will call "RD" in the interview below) from Columbia, who attended the University of South Carolina. Her father was a root doctor. She spoke of his ability to "turn it [the curse] back on the root doctor who had sent it by returning the offending root to the root doctor's property or by simply casting the spell back through his power of concentration and projection of mental energy." She described an incident where the offending root doctor actually appeared on their doorstep one day and asked her father to take his own original curse off him. It appears that he had recognized the physical and psychic signs of the reversal, and through the community, learned which root doctor had turned it back on him. This young woman's father was, like many other root doctors, a devout Christian. He therefore made the afflicted root doctor swear to stop casting evil roots before agreeing to release him from the one under which he was currently suffering.

Sheriff McTeer recounted a similar conclusion to a psychic war he had with the famous Doctor Buzzard. McTeer ordered Dr. Buzzard to stop selling potions. This particular war of curse and counter-curses ended with the drowning death of Dr. Buzzard's son. Soon after, Dr Buzzard visited McTeer and the two men made peace and became friends of a sort.

Over the years, on several occasions I have been asked to magically help a client cause harm to someone. I usually refuse outright and try to reason with the person to use other ways of dealing with their anger and fear. On one occasion in 2005, however, I conducted a spiritual healing ritual for an old friend in middle Tennessee. The healing appeared to provide some relief from a painful debilitating nerve disorder. At the end of the ritual, my friend, a late middle-aged woman, asked me to create a root or magical device for the purpose of hurting a man by whom she felt threatened.

I asked her, "Are you sure this is what you want? Remember that things you do will eventually find their way back to you." She seemed adamant in her assertions and intent, so I opened my box of magical ingredients and prepared a root containing goofer-dust, a lodestone for energy and other herbal ingredients traditionally designed to cause harm. After charging it, I handed it to her and told her to keep it in a secure place. When she needed to inflict harm on this person, she was to visualize him and squeeze the charm with all her might. She seemed satisfied and we soon left for the drive back to Kentucky.

On the way home, my wife asked me, "What do you think she'll do?"

I replied that she was basically a kind, decent person who was just hurting and afraid. "Just wait and see!" I replied. "I believe that once she thinks about what she is doing, she will reconsider."

About two weeks later, the same woman telephoned and asked if she could get rid of the root because she "did not like having it around anymore." I told her to bury it in a place sacred to her. This woman practices Native American spirituality and is a gifted psychic, so I am sure that upon reflection, she remembered, that to intentionally inflict harm on another is to harm one's self and those you love as well. Fear and anger, while powerful motivators, tend to make a person reckless and prone to seek immediate answers. Fear also empowers the person causing the harm. It also betrays a lack of faith in one's own abilities and faith in the Divine's overall plan and our part in it. As Lee Gandee would say "Your fear and your anger is your worst enemy in magic. Calm down, and think before you strike."

The third magical skill expected of a root doctor is the ability to provide magical protection for his or her clients. This is performed through rituals and/or the creation of charms that would provide protection, provide luck, gain the affections of another, win at games of chance, win in a legal matter or a host of other needs, limited only by the patient's desires and ability to compensate the root doctor. Names for these types of protective amulets are many, including mojo bags, Tobies, tricks or roots. The root doctor might supply a simple amulet for the person to wear or hang in the home. Additional magical protection may be to provide a mixture of herbs and powders with which to bathe or wash the floors and walls to magically cleanse a dwelling.

The actual formulas for these charms are as varied as the practitioners who create them; however, certain rules are generally followed. For example, the symbolism of color is fairly consistently employed, with blue for love, green for money, black for harm and red for protection. Red flannel is the most common packaging medium for the ingredients of a protective charm/root. Its historical use is traceable to the African, Caribbean and European magical traditions. Newbell Niles Puckett in his study of Hoodoo charms, *Folk Beliefs of the Southern Negro* said, "In both Europe and Africa it may well be that the red color represents what was formerly sacrificial blood offered to the fetish in question" (221). A charm may be a complex mixture of ingredients or may take a form as simple as wearing a piece of sliver as a disrupter of negative energy. In the past, a silver dime was often worn as an amulet tied to the ankle with a piece of red string.

As stated above, often a root will contain a biological product like animal bones, teeth, or human blood, semen, hair, or fingernails. These personal items are included to tie the effect of the charm to a certain individual. Personalization of the charm is critical to the casting of the spell. A love charm often might contain some part of the intended lover's person or some part of the person casting the spell. Menstrual blood was a commonly used component in charms for women in hopes of securing the affections of a lover. With the modern threat of diseases like AIDS, the popular use of such products has waned but not disappeared. I once observed the creation and charging of a charm that was to be used to reinvigorate a husband's sexual ability, which, for some reason, had lost the required vigor and stamina. The charm contained a wax image with a wooden phallus and the man's pubic hair to personalize the charm, which was then wrapped in a red flannel sheath. His wife then added a bit of her own personal lubrication to ensure that when invigorated, his abilities would remain focused toward her. The charm was then placed in the mattress underneath where the man slept as a sort of magical Viagra. As was later reported to me, the charm had produced the desired effect, in abundance!

Where there's a need, there's merchandizing!

This need for certain supplies in creation of these charms led to the commercialization of the Hoodoo charm and the creation of an entire network of suppliers and distributors. Long traces the beginnings of this unique American enterprise from its roots in the early 1900s, through their heyday in the 1920s and 1930s, to their modern manifestations. These businesses are still economically viable and have been invigorated by the influx of individuals from the Caribbean and South America. According to Long, the "spiritual products industry is evolving and expanding" (249).

I remember asking the Beaufort root doctor and sheriff, James McTeer, about the commercially produced materials and the need to go foraging in the woods for the herbs, roots and other naturally occurring items needed to prepare the charms or roots needed in their practice. He readily acknowledged that he and most of the root doctors he knew no longer foraged the woods and swamps for their magical supplies, but purchased them from supply houses from as far away as Chicago and New York.

A final traditional role expected of the root doctor was the ability to communicate with the unseen world of spirits and other forces that affected the lives of their clients. The world of spirits is routinely consulted during the diagnosis phase of the treatment of an illness. This is because the spirits are not bound by physical form and are witness and privy to information outside the range of the embodied. Spirit communication can be employed for diagnosing the source of an illness or locating the whereabouts of a missing person or thing. Communication with the spirit world often involves entering a deep trance state. The root doctor's skill of projecting his own spirit or consciousness into this unseen realm for purposes of spirit communication is related to the widespread Low Country belief that each human is in possession of two souls—or two aspects of the same soul—depending on who you interview. In their article "The Gullah Language and Sea Island Culture," Dennis Adams and Hillary Barnwell describe a process of soul division: "the 'soul' leaves the body and returns to God at death, but the 'spirit'

stays on earth—still involved in the daily affairs of its living descendants."
Such a metaphysical belief also creates the need for honoring one's ancestors.
As a result, formal mourning rituals are conducted and burial practices are
elaborate, often involving grave decoration, which include broken household
items and natural substances, like seashells, which symbolize "the belief that
the dead reside in a realm beneath river bottoms" ("Religion" 1).

Many of the activities of the root doctor are conducted while in a state
of light to moderate trance. One root doctor described the trance process
as being between asleep and being awake. In this enhanced state of awareness, spirits appear to the root doctor according to his or her state of mind.
"You'd better be in the right frame of mind when you deal with spirits,"
one elderly woman from Georgetown, South Carolina advised me, "If you
aren't, they (the spirits) can sure mess you up!" Clearly, spirit communication is not a game, an experiment or a process to be taken lightly. Most
root doctors have a single spirit or a select few entities that they trust and
from whom they will accept information. Sometimes the spirit is a trusted
relative who has died.

I had a conversation with the young female informant noted above
("RD"—the daughter of a root doctor, and, I believe, his successor) about
her family's experiences with spirit contacts:

RD: My Daddy always talks to his mother! She is always in our home and
      I've seen her, too.

JM: When do you see her?

RD: Daddy taught me how to see her. You relax, close your eyes, but not
      all the way, and let your mind empty and then think about her. After
      a while, things begin to look different.

JM: In what way?

RD: It just does, not like regular life. The room looks the same, but it's
      like a curtain is lifted and there's more there than you normally see.
      Pretty soon, Grandma comes in, just like when she was living. She
      always looks happy and smiles.

JM: Does she talk to you?

RD: Not like you and I are now. She talks to you in your mind.

JM: Can she touch you?

RD: Yes, of course! I even feel her touch me when I can't see her. She even saved me from being badly hurt one time.

JM: How?

RD: I was out riding one Saturday with some friends. . . . Everybody was drinking, you know. All of a sudden, I felt Grandma grab my arm and heard her say in my ear "Get out of this car!" Nobody else heard her. I made them stop and let me out at my house. They all thought I was crazy, but later that night they were all in a bad wreck.

JM: Incredible! Did you know your Grandma before she passed away?

RD: I was small when she died, but I remember her. I love her being around now, it makes me feel safe.

Above everything else, the spirits of the dead must be treated with respect and appeased when they are angry or disturbed. The living must secure ways to communicate with these spirits, and the root doctor is the vehicle for that communication. One additional expectation is that the root doctor can also summon and employ certain spirits to do his or her bidding in some magical matter. The use of graveyard dirt in a charm is done to secure the services of the spirit by binding that spirit to that charm and spell. The root doctor will seek the grave dirt of an individual who has been executed, done grave harm in life or committed suicide, because that spirit is trapped between the worlds and may be desperate to make amends to God for his transgressions as an embodied person. Sometimes, however, a magical intrusion stems from the attack of an evil or rogue spirit such as the famous "plat-eye." E. Randall Floyd, in the *Augusta Chronicle Online*, describes it "as a much-feared spirit that supposedly haunted and tormented its victims unmercifully before driving them either to insane asylums or early graves" and adds

> According to legends probably brought over from Europe, plat-eyes were evil spirits that came back to life for one of several reasons to avenge their deaths, to cause mischief among mortals, or to finish up tasks begun in life. Failure to provide the departed with a proper burial was also a good way to warrant an unwelcome visit by the plat-eye. (1)

As we can see, the fear of the plat-eye was tied to traditional beliefs in the spirits of the ancestors and the observance of proper funeral customs. One young woman from Orangeburg, South Carolina, told me that you could not normally see a plat-eye but, if you were unlucky, feel its presence on lonely stretches of road near rural cemeteries. She said, "When I pass a cemetery at night by myself, I say the Lord's Prayer and hit the gas pedal!"

Another common manifestation of spirit attack is called being "hag ridden." In this situation, a spirit or shape-shifting witch has projected their consciousness into victim's bedroom and attacked them by sitting on the victim's chest while hitting, biting, scratching or slapping the victim, leaving them feeling dreadful and exhausted in the morning. As in our earlier examples, additional signs of attack by a spirit or "haint" include finding a person in an unresponsive or trance-like state. It can also appear as a sudden change in habits and personality or persistent and intense nightmares that leave physical signs, such as unexplained scratches and bruises. Such evidence indicates that a conventional doctor must first be consulted and then in the absence of any natural cause, a root doctor should be sought without delay. A person can also protect himself or herself from being hag-ridden by placing certain charms on the bedpost, putting salt on the open windowsill or placing a large piece of iron under the bed to act as a barrier to the psychic energy. Such an evil or rogue spirit can also be trapped by the root doctor in a jug or bottle and thereby rendered harmless. Cornelia Walker Bailey, Low Country author of *God, Dr. Buzzard and the Bolito Man,* describes the process of trapping the hag:

But there was only one way you could stop the hag from visiting altogether. You could put salt in an open bottle and leave it near the bed and the hag would fly into that bottle with the salt. The salt would hold her there and she couldn't get out. In the morning, you'd put a cap on the bottle and you'd say. "I gotcha now" and you could actually hear the hag screaming in the bottle, "let me out, let me out." You buried the bottle in the ground then the hag wouldn't bother you no more. (142)

I was once shown a bottle by Lee Gandee in the Dutch Fork of South Carolina that was said to have been imprisoning an evil spirit for more than a hundred years. It was clouded and had salt and hair woven inside the neck of the bottle. When asked if I'd like to be the one to open the bottle, I respectfully declined.

The Root Doctor's Magic: What Is It and How Does It Work?

All shamans, whether root doctors, powwows or grannies, practice the same essential types of magic, which are:

Sympathetic magic

The 19th-century anthropologist James Gordon Frazer, in his famous work, *The Golden Bough*, defines the principle of sympathetic magic as "that like produces like, or that an effect resembles its cause" ("Sympathetic" 1). This magical practice has its roots in what he calls the Law of Similarity. Frazer says the "magician infers that he can produce any effect he desires merely by imitating it" ("Sympathetic" 1). An example in Hoodoo practice would be the casting of a spell upon an object that has been constructed to resemble or otherwise symbolically represent the person. A wax or wooden image of a person is dressed in certain colors and is anointed with certain powders, oils or symbols as the spell is cast. If the doll were to contain hair or other items owned by or physically related to the person, the additional element of contagious magic would be brought into play.

One classic charm, from the famous Madam Collins of Memphis, would allow a woman to control her lover's potency so that unless he was with her, he could not perform and would "lose his nature." Carolyn Morrow Long records in *Spiritual Merchants: Religion, Magic and Commerce* that the recipe required the use of a cloth or length of cord with which she was "to wipe the semen from her lover's penis after intercourse, tie the cloth in nine knots and wear it next to her skin or hidden in her mattress" (87). This particular version of sympathetic magic is called homeopathic magic, or the use of small portions of a thing to represent and affect the intended object of the magic. A specially prepared image, often containing some physical possession or personal element like hair, fingernails or skin of a person may be manipulated in some manner in the belief that actions taken on this substitute will then have an effect of the intended person. A well-known modern example of this magical practice is the desecration and burning of an effigy of a hated person, despised political figure or even a dummy figure from rival sports team. Although most modern people would, upon being questioned, would never admit or acknowledge the magical process involved, they will still invest great time and energy in such a magically focused event. Imitation of the action desired is the key to this sort of magical practice. Even today, women who wish to bear children will travel to the Dorset countryside and lightheartedly sit upon the huge phallus of the 180-foot-tall Cerne Abbas Giant, which is carved into the hillside where chalk deposits lie right beneath the surface of the land. Dancing around the festive maypole on May Day has long been recognized as a survival of an old rite of fertility and a form of sympathetic magic.

Contagious magic

The second major type of magic is called contagious magic. Frazer defines contagious magic as the belief that "things which have once been conjoined must remain ever afterwards, even when quite dissevered from each other, in such a sympathetic relation that whatever is done to the one must similarly affect the other" ("Contagious"1). In this practice, there exists a belief in an interconnected relationship between all people and things in the universe. A good example of contagious magic would be the casting of a spell by placing a charm or powder where the intended recipient will come into contact with it and be affected. The famous root doctor, Dr Buzzard, of St. Helena Island, South Carolina, was known for spreading powder in the courtroom before a criminal or civil trial to affect those who would come into contact with or see it rendering them unable to give evidence as a witness and, I suspect, to influence the jury as well. Another common technique employed in contagious magic would be for the root doctor to bury a root somewhere inside the house or on the property of the intended victim. Often people would report feeling a sudden pain as they passed over the object. This was an indication of the presence of a malevolent spell, which is actually a form of magical poisoning. As a young root doctor from Columbia, South Carolina, said, "When I was young, my grandfather [also a root doctor] would bury a root out by the back porch where the person he was after would be sure to step on it. Once he did, that was it!"

Famous Carolina Root Doctors

Reminiscent of their African counterparts, root doctors in the Low Country would often assume a name that symbolized their particular practice or personality. Three of the most famous traditional root doctors of the coastal Carolina area took the names of birds or insects; hence, there were names like Dr. Hawk, Dr. Bug, Dr. Eagle, Dr. Snake, Dr. Crow and the most famous of all, Dr. Buzzard. Many operated out of rented space or from their homes, like Dr. Eagle (born P.C. Washington), who was remarkable for his deep, piercing eyes. Many had other sources of income, like Dr. Hawk, who ran his own grocery store.

Most of the old time root doctors were recognized early in their lives as having a special personal quality that gave them access to the world of spirits and the ability to heal. It is widely believed that a child who is born with a caul or membrane over the face at birth has been chosen by the spirit world for a special role in life. The survival from a dangerous accident or a miraculous recovery from a near-fatal illness can bestow such a spiritual mantle. In these cases, the living soul has passed temporarily into the spirit realm and returned to this existence, bringing back some of the otherworldly presence. Being born with a particularly dark complexion was thought to confer special powers for working magic or communicating with the spirit world.

In her memoir, *God, Dr. Buzzard and the Bolito Man: A Saltwater Geechee Talks about Life on Sapelo Island, Georgia,* Cornelia Walker Bailey recalls a powerful female root doctor she calls "Mama Lizzie." Mama Lizzie was not a community healer but someone you consulted when you wanted "to put an evil spell on somebody" (Bailey 191). Known for her cruelty, vindictiveness and short temper, Mama Lizzie was feared and respected throughout the island community, regardless of educational level or position in life. Bailey recounts how an affront to one of Mama Lizzie's sisters was handled by magically and fatally poisoning the offender. Bailey recalls, "One of the things I've learned from living on a small island where our roots have been for two hundred years is that our traditions get passed down, yes, but so do our hurts and angers. They get handed down from generation to generation" (194).

The legendary "Doctor Buzzard"

Little is known of the early life of the most famous South Carolina Low Country root doctor of modern times, "Dr. Buzzard," who was said to "be as powerful as a buzzard and to have the patience of a buzzard" (Bailey 190). He was born Stephaney Robinson, lived and operated on St. Helena Island where his power and influence became unrivaled. Root doctor and high sheriff James McTeer said that Dr. Buzzard was particularly adept at "chewing the root" in court. He would simply sit in the court, behind his purple sunglasses, staring at the proposed witness. The effect was devastating to a prosecuting attorney, who found he had a witness who had become completely incapable of giving testimony.

"Chewing the root" is a powerful form of spell-casting, which is witnessed by the intended victim and usually others nearby. "Chewing the root" demonstrates the two facets of the root doctor's spell-casting. The first concerns the personal magical power he or she can summon and the ability to focus that power externally with intention and tangibility. The second involves the public practice of that magical power, where it is witnessed and understood by the victim and the community. This action creates and enhances the personal reputation of the root doctor if the spell is deemed to be effective and the perception of his or her power becomes a part of the collective perception of reality for the community.

Roger Pinckney, in *Blue Roots: African-American Folk Magic of the Gullah People,* describes how "a root doctor makes up a root, tracks down his victim and chews it in his presence all the while making signs and speaking in unknown tongues" (indicating a possible state of trance). "The effect is terrifying—the doctor swaying, muttering, eyes rolled back in his head, juice from the root running down his chin. . . . , often bringing the victim to his knees" (Pinckney 54).

It is important to note that in Hoodoo, a spell or root can be delivered through the eyes or the voice. The concept behind this projection centers on the belief that the power of the soul can be seen and witnessed and hence projected through the eyes and voice. The life-energy of a person's will has the ability to travel in this manner to wherever it is directed. This concept is at the heart of shamanic spell-casting. The practice of projection transcends cultures.

Some readers will invariably ask, "But is this really happening? Can they really do that?" To answer these questions, we must examine our own perception of reality, which is largely the result of an unconscious, collective agreement as to what our reality is at this moment in history.

All cultures are in a constant process of defining their collective reality, based on current evidence and the information they receive as an ongoing process of being self-aware, embodied entities. A person's perception of reality is also impacted by the claims of the socially dominant group. As we have seen in the colonial period, the socially dominant group determined that those without power and wealth deserved to be viewed as inferior and deserved social exploitation. That perception of reality became the lens through which they saw the world, other human beings and life in general. Like all cultures, they formulated and codified their beliefs, designed tests to verify them and drew up the psychological and perceptive boundaries of their worldview. The concept of shamanic projection of personal energy is a perfect example of an idea that exists outside our modern worldview and collective perception of reality. To assert the existence of this idea is a threat to the collective mindset. We must therefore expect it to be challenged and attacked. Small wonder such thinking exists at the social boundaries of our culture and are thought of as the beliefs of a marginal group of people. Those for whom such ideas are a reality or who have been affected by these practices are considered deluded or deceived. Yet even our modern culture of scientific rationalism will suspend its collective social dominance and critical assessment of its worldview to accommodate the beliefs of conventional, socially accepted religious practices and beliefs no matter how similar or fantastic those beliefs may appear to be. The reality of projection and magical practice in general seems to peck at the walls of that conventional worldview, offering a hint at just what might exist beyond its gates.

Sometimes the root doctor's name became his or hers as an inheritance or by appropriation, as with Dr. Buzzard, who took his name from an earlier Caucasian root doctor. This earlier root doctor, according to Henry Middleton Hyatt, died around the turn of the last century (1414, 1418).

The modern Dr. Buzzard, like most root doctors, charged for his services and potions, and became quite wealthy in the process. As large numbers of African Americans moved to Northern cities, taking their beliefs and customs like spiritual baggage, root doctors like Dr. Buzzard often served these clients via telephone calls and the postal service. Dr. Buzzard, like many of his counterparts, was extremely knowledgeable and careful of the laws surrounding the sale of "homemade medicines." My informant told me that Dr. Buzzard, realizing that to cash his money orders would require his signature and hence incriminate him, stood in the post office and ripped to pieces more than ten thousand dollars' worth of postal money orders.

Pinckney illustrates a valid and ironic paradox of the struggle between the traditional healer, the legal system and medical profession when he says,

> There is no law in South Carolina against the removing of spells or against the casting of them even if such hexes result in disability and death. But if a root doctor gives a client a salve, a body oil or any potion to be taken internally, he can be cited for 'practicing medicine without a license' regardless of how effective or benign the substance might be. (50)

Pinckney's statement also reflects the professional territoriality and social perception of root doctors and other non-traditional healers who operate outside the culture of scientific rationalism. To prosecute a person for casting or removing a spell would be to acknowledge that it exists. Without that acknowledgment, no matter the cost, it can simply be ignored and derided as superstitious nonsense.

Stephaney Robinson, Dr. Buzzard, died in 1947. His earthly remains reside in an unmarked grave, the location of which is kept a closely guarded secret to this day, to prevent grave desecration, as the bones of one so revered and feared would have great magical and monetary value.

Other root doctors, in their zeal or greed were not as careful as Dr. Buzzard and occasionally ran afoul of the law. In his autobiography, *High Sheriff of the Low-country,* J.E. McTeer gives an account of the exploits of "Dr. Bug" during the Second World War. Dr. Bug (Peter Murray) was not a typical root doctor but was apparently an enterprising individual who saw an opportunity and took it. Without training, he set himself up in practice, selling potions to young men who wished to evade the draft. McTeer says,

"Dozens of young colored [sic] men were being rejected at their pre-induction physicals and were coming home classified 4-F" (24). This brought about a police and FBI investigation, which uncovered that Dr. Bug had been supplying these young men with an arsenic-laced potion that could have killed them if they'd taken too much. Dr. Bug lost his practice and went to prison for his carelessness and greed.

I must not give the impression that root doctors are limited to the South Carolina Low Country. The root doctor is not just a rural phenomenon but, according to Dr. Hazel Weidman, who studied the practice and clinical treatment in Miami in the 1970s, "You'll find root work of one form or another in any urban area of the country that has a large black population" (qtd. in Michaelson 39). Root doctors have appeared wherever African Americans and many Southern whites lived and needed their services. In Newport, Arkansas, Aunt Caroline Dye was widely known for the efficacy of her cures, charms and her ability to commune with spirit forces. In his excellent biography, *The Fabled Doctor Jim Jordan: A Story of Conjure*, Roy Johnson details the life of a conjure doctor in the Murfreesboro area of North Carolina. Jordan had a shamanistic career that spanned almost fifty years, and he was known far beyond the boundaries of his community. Born to parents who had been slaves, Jordan claimed that his knowledge had its roots with the practices of the local Native Americans. There are local accounts from the 1700s of Indian chiefs sending for African American slave-healers when illness struck. This strongly indicates ongoing social contact and the presence of trained healers and spirit shamans among the slave population.

Jordan, like so many of his counterparts in the Carolinas and Georgia, openly professed that his power and practice were an enhancement of his Christian faith, yet, according to Johnson, many in his community continued "harboring dark fear of the mysterious workings of the spirit world [and] would not abandon suspicion he abstained completely from black magic" (1).

Jim Jordan's personal story is typical of many root doctors. His childhood was steeped in local traditions and lore, including, Johnson notes in his biography, the presence of anti-theft charms like "blue bottles containing an assortment of things hanging from a white lady's peach trees" (36). First, hanging the charm bottles in the tree was the magical work of a "white lady," indicating the prevalence and exchange of magical practices between both races. The use of "witch bottles" is traceable to its origins in the British Isles. Second, the fact that such a sight was easily recognized and interpreted by members of the African American community is indicative of significant social interaction and a commonality of this type of symbolism. The use of bottles, pots and other containers for magical purpose also is traceable to the African subcontinent.

Jordan learned much of his practice, which included herb- and spirit-based remedies, from an uncle who was a well known conjure doctor. Like many of his contemporaries, he attended school and had a very basic education, meaning he could read and write. Upon his uncle's death, Jordan took over his practice and quickly became well known and patronized. It is important to note that his magical practice was, for most of his life, a lucrative sideline, while he managed a successful farming and logging business with his sons. Caught ill-prepared for the farm reforms of the 1950s, Johnson says, "Jordan's conjure business saved him from bankruptcy" (119). It is for his magical practice and his civic generosity that James Jordan is remembered to this day. Upon his death in 1962, his status as a physical, psychological and spiritual healer had reached legendary proportions. His life story illustrates that, as often as not, the root doctor was a productive and respected member of the community, who was, in addition to his magical practice, also immersed in the ordinary life of the community as well.

The Darker Side of Conjure

As noted earlier, most root doctors and healers demonstrate some ability or aptitude for this work as children and were and are groomed for their work. Some, like a grandmotherly woman from Georgetown, were healers with a singular ability to correct one type of injury or illness. This woman had the ability to "talk the fire" or heal burned skin. Not only would the pain vanish, but often, no trace of the burn would remain after her "treatment." It must be stated that most of these people profess themselves to be good Christians and considered the healing work "a calling" from the Divine. "It's all a blessing from the Lord!" the healer from Georgetown would remind me. "I can do this because God says so, not because I say so." On the other hand, there were other individuals who took on the more suspect role of conversing with the dead, which was always seen as walking a thin line between good and evil. There were also those who become enamored with the power they have and decide at some point to, use their magic and powers to cause harm.

During my fieldwork, I learned of a very powerful, but ruthless root doctor from down on the Georgia coast. This man held an entire community in his power and tolerated no challenge to his dominance. Once, when challenged by another conjure woman, the old root doctor somehow caused her house to burn, killing her child. The local minister chose the boy's funeral to deliver a fiery denouncement of witchcraft and root doctors. As the congregation arrived at the small rural church the next Sunday, they were greeted by a gruesome response from the root doctor. On the steps of the church, attached to the top of a pole was the decapitated head of the little boy buried just the week before. The message was clear, and no further challenges were heard in that small rural community. No police were summoned, no charges filed. This story is not designed to titillate but to illustrate the fact that this type of activity was and is not a parlor game but a deadly serious business.

If a root doctor magically caused someone's death, no police would interfere, but the community might decide that his presence could no longer be tolerated. While doing my initial fieldwork in the mid-1970s, on my way to class, I would often pass a small house in downtown Columbia, within a mile of the USC campus and state capitol. The house was unmistakably marked as the home of a root doctor. Upon investigation, I learned that, indeed, a root doctor had taken up residence there and was considered to be a dangerous person, capable of anything. One afternoon as I passed by, I noticed that the house had been magically neutralized. When I asked what had become of the individual who lived there, I was told that he had met with a sudden tragic accident and that his presence would not be missed. I was advised to ask no more questions and to not mention the person or the incident again. It was made clear to me that what had happened was "for the best."

It may be difficult for many people today to understand the persistence of such beliefs and to conceive of how such things could happen in an age of mass media and the scientific-rational paradigms of modern society.

Please remember that the culture of the root doctor remains a publicly unacknowledged and invisible culture that operates seamlessly in modern life by its own set of rules, ethics and unique perception of reality. It is immune to the incursions of education, social position and outside indoctrination, because it lives in a deep part of the psyches of the people who have, even subconsciously, embraced it through their upbringing or beliefs. James McTeer once told me, "Everyone has a belief in this, somewhere in their minds. You may not think you believe in magic, but somewhere in your mind, you do. That's the part of your mind I can reach when I put a spell on you. It's the part of your mind you can't control, like your dreams, and the more you deny it, the stronger it grows."

The Ongoing Social Encounter and Impact of Hoodoo

Today, many medical and law enforcement professionals do not recognize the signs and signals of a culture that has had centuries of practice in being invisible. Even if they do recognize the signs and make inquiries, they will most likely learn nothing or be fed misinformation. If, for example, a person is found dead under peculiar circumstances or wastes away in a hospital for no apparent cause, basic inquiries are made, nothing is learned and the case goes unsolved. Remember that for most of its history, official representatives of the government have treated such beliefs with scorn and contempt, further disenfranchising those people and their beliefs from the mainstream culture. As a result of this cultural alienation, these "official" opinions and ideas carry no weight or authority within the Hoodoo community. Local politicians and upwardly mobile people of the community often publicly deny the existence of a magical culture in their backyard. They fear their community will appear socially backward and that community investment from the outside will be negatively impacted.

Regardless of these attempts to hide the presence and ongoing belief in Hoodoo, many conventional medical practitioners will continue to encounter people and illnesses that reflect these unique beliefs and practices. Many physicians have learned the wisdom of treating such beliefs with respect and working with the patient within the context of those beliefs, which constitute his or her personal reality. Some mental health therapists have employed shamanistic techniques successfully when treating patients with certain disorders. Many conventional physicians in the Carolina Low Country, like Dr. Edward McNeil and Dr. LaFrance Ferguson, medical director at Beaufort-Jasper-Hampton Comprehensive Health Services Inc., have learned that the medical aspects of Hoodoo and root working are worthy of consideration. This is indicated in the following passage by Will Dean from "Hoodoo Medicine in the Lowcountry," which appeared in the March 7, 2004, online news magazine *Lowcountry NOW*:

> When she started with the organization more than 16 years ago, Ferguson's patients would tell her about placing moss in shoes to lower high blood pressure, and using garlic and other unconventional remedies. "Now they're talking more about medications," she said.
>
> Ferguson's reaction, then and now, is to listen. "I was pretty accepting of the beliefs unless I knew it was something that was totally going to cause them some harm. It made them more amendable to using my methods," she said.
>
> "I was open to hearing them and I did not find them odd and I did not demean them. Sometimes as clinicians we don't know everything scientifically."
>
> Dr. Edward McNeil, who has practiced medicine in Beaufort County since 1983, agrees it's a mistake for physicians "to dismiss Gullah medical practices . . ." "Some of what (Gullah) people do is some of what we do," he said. "A lot of these roots and things could have medications. Some roots have diuretics. The problem is the quantification and purification. They might take more or less than the day before.
>
> "What we do is more scientific, (but) the soul is involved in healing as well as the spirit," he said. (1)

Recently, Hoodoo, as a magical practice has enjoyed a modern revival via the Internet and through the efforts of many teacher-practitioners, such as noted Hoodoo authority and practitioner, Catherine Yronwode of Forestville, California. Yronwode maintains an extensive website containing many informational articles and a spiritual supply house called the Lucky Mojo Curio Company, which sells all the spiritual products needed, from High John Conqueror root for protection to raccoon penis bones for success in gambling. She has published her own excellent book on Hoodoo and teaches an online course in how to practice this magical art. Yronwode is one of many modern proponents of Hoodoo. Augustine's Spiritual Goods located in Hancock, Michigan, is owned and operated by "Rev. Frank PaPa Doc" and "Miss Alice," who sell a wide variety of products and services, including "Dr. Buzzard's Court Case Powder and Court Case Oil" which draws on the legendary powers of the Beaufort, South Carolina, Dr. Buzzard's ability to affect the outcome of legal proceedings. Many modern root doctors also discreetly advertise themselves in spiritual magazines and even in the classified sections of local newspapers. It has become clear during the writing of this book that even though still basically invisible to the general public, the practice of Hoodoo is still alive and very healthy in this first decade of the twenty-first century. Traditional magical practice remains a relevant and powerful force in the lives of many modern Americans.

CHAPTER TWO

Interview
James E. McTeer, the "White Prince"

You can only perceive real beauty in a person as they get older.
—Anouk Aimee, O *Magazine,* October 2003

Wisdom outweighs any wealth.   —Sophocles, *Antigone*

I SUCCEEDED in locating my first actual contact to the unique and hidden world of Hoodoo and root doctor practice on a tip from a classmate from the South Carolina Low Country. The man I was introduced to was known as the "White Prince"—Mr. James E. McTeer, root doctor and former sheriff of Beaufort, South Carolina.

During the course of my research in the mid-1970s, I conducted interviews with a number of people involved in the Hoodoo tradition, both white and African American. After those initial college papers were written, all the tapes, along with the field notes went into boxes and a suitcase where they languished for almost thirty years. During those years, tapes were lost, damaged and copied over. As a result, this one interview with James McTeer is the only complete tape to have survived intact.

When I first met James E. McTeer, he was a retired high sheriff who, in 1974, operated a small real estate company in the coastal area of Beaufort, South Carolina. At our initial contact, I found him to be a genteel, educated man with a powerful presence that had not diminished with age. His personality was adequately reflected in the inscription on the James E. McTeer Bridge, where he is described as a "legendary lawman, author, spellbinder and raconteur." As we talked in his office he told me how he had been born to a traditional, Low Country plantation family, and as such, grew up in a world of myth, magic and legend. Hoodoo and root doctoring were as common as the Spanish moss that hangs from trees just about everywhere in Beaufort County.

His eventual adoption of a root doctor's mantle allowed him, as a sheriff and a white person, to penetrate areas of his community otherwise unavailable and unseen to the casual observer. His practice had continued even after he retired from his professional life.

"I've been trying to retire for five years!" he exclaimed and added that the demand for his services was still too great. He often referred to himself as a "poor man's psychiatrist," meaning that he realized that he provided some level of counseling to those who could not afford or who distrusted conventional therapists. His acknowledged role as a counselor, however, did not mean that he thought that magic was all in a person's mind or just the power of suggestion.

In his book, High Sheriff of the Low Country, McTeer chronicled how, in 1926 at age 22, he became one of the nation's youngest high sheriffs. During his 37-year career in Beaufort County, South Carolina, he dealt with everything from major crimes to smuggling to Nazi submarines to a nudist colony.

According to McTeer, the mind is a tool, which can be honed to an advanced state of awareness, capable of sensing the unseen, projecting the consciousness and affecting the material world.

When "clients" would arrive, they would be taken to the back room and seated on a chair facing the altar. Most of the time, after consultation, McTeer would usually lay hands upon the person and chant the appropriate spell.

Like other root doctors I encountered, McTeer's powers of concentration were incredible in their intensity, often resembling a state of deep trance. It was at this point that they "had the power" to perform the task required of them. I usually sat nearby, after having been introduced as an apprentice from out of town. Once, during one of these sessions, McTeer's hands accidentally brushed my shoulder as he passed them over his client. The effect was like being jolted by an electric current and left me dazed for several minutes.

Here is a sample of a typical field interview, which was conducted in 1974 in his real estate office in downtown Beaufort, South Carolina. The people involved are me (JM), McTeer (McT) and Jan, a friend who came with me on this interview.

(*Author's Note:* Most of the following is dialogue, but there are occasional breaks in the interviews to include brief incidental information. As an aside, Mr. McTeer often used the term "witchdoctor" to describe himself.)

McT: I've been trying to retire from witchcraft for five years.

JM: Let me ask you something; Most of the people who come to you, are they suffering from some sort of psychosomatic illness? What would you do if you realized they had a physical illness? Would you send them to a regular doctor?

McT: Oh, indeed I do! I say, "This is a physical illness, that arthritis, that goiter, that tumor has nothing to do with witchcraft," and I beseech them to go on to their doctors. What I treat is to cure their mental illness and magical illnesses. I am the best friend the doctor's got! I don't pretend to be able to cure high blood pressure, except to relieve them of their worries.

JM: I read that this is where the old witchdoctors got into trouble by trying to cure everything. I read about Dr. Bug in the article by the Charleston psychiatrist, Ramsey Mellette.

McT: I taught Dr. Mellette right on the couch where you are sitting. Dr. Mellette came in for three lectures by me and I'll tell you my lectures are long. I trained Dr. Mellette. I coined the term "poor man's psychiatrist."

JM: Is anyone still living?

I was referring to an earlier interview topic about the old-time root doctors.

McT: Hawk is dead, Eagle is dead, Bug is dead, Buzzard is dead. . . . All of them had counterparts, but they don't have the *savior faire* that those old witchdoctors had. They were the true descendants of the African witchdoctors, and now their sons-in-law have taken over and they're just opportunists.

JM: You mentioned during another interview that what it [root doctoring] was all about now was the opportunists.

McT: That's right! Like that Anton LeVey, the Satanist—I have dozens of women come here. They come here four and five in a big Cadillac car and ask me "We want you to form us a coven!" And if you do that, why there'll be other covens that will be formed. I tell them there's no chance in the world. I don't believe in covens. They are searching for something new, something to occupy themselves. . . . Then they all get together naked and hold hands in a circle. It's all a show!

JM: A new name for the same old thing!

McT: That's right!

JM: Has there ever been a case of a Zombie in this area?

McT: The Zombie is associated with Voodoo in Haiti, Santo Domingo. Zombie is bringing the dead back to life. Never! Here we have the Evil Eye, putting a spell on you and having a witchdoctor project himself into your home at night, project himself into your bedroom and take possession of your mind. That's what happens! Projection!

JM: Is most of the Hoodoo that is practiced now on the medicine (healing) end of things or on the magical side?

McT: I know positively that I have saved three people from suicide in the past three months. People who came here for a cure as a last result. They had spells on them and a sickness had been cast against them and they had given up. They were going to commit suicide and wanted to see me before they did it because they had heard about me. I talked them out of it. Last week I had a doctor call me up and said he had a black girl who was supposed to go in the hospital to have a baby and the baby was going to be one of these hard deliveries. There was going be serious trouble and chances are it would be a cesarean. She had got to the [hospital] door and said, "No, I can't come in the hospital." She had a spell on her and she was told that if she went into the hospital, she'd die. So they sent her to me and had me take that spell off her. I took it off her; she went into the hospital and lived. You have no idea of the scope of it [Hoodoo] and the size of it. I average three to five telephone calls a week from California, Las Vegas, Seattle, Washington, Pittsburgh—

There was a knock at the door.

McT: Come in!

A former client arrived. Mr. McTeer and the client adjourned to the back room where the altar was, spoke for a few minutes and then the client left.

JM: You mentioned before that this girl was black. Would you say that the belief or the influence of it [Hoodoo] is mostly in the black population?

McT: Oh, it's seventy-five percent white now! Oh yes, it's preponderantly white.

JM: Are most of them educated? Formally?

McT: Well, let's see this right here.

He showed me a letter asking for magical help written by a client on the business letterhead from a major corporation in the urban, northeastern part of the country.

McT: I have college professors coming here. I have men who are flying Harrier [military] airplanes come here who are under some spell.

He then handed me another recent letter pleading for help.

JM: She wants her husband to come back to her.

McT: I get these sorts of things all the time.

My friend Jan was reading some of McTeer's letters and notes as he and I talked.

Jan: Look here! You wanted to know about the plat-eye, here's a letter here from Washington, D.C.

McT: That came in during the last two weeks.

Jan: Whew! Good grief, he has been in such agony, it's pitiful. . . . There he is!

She showed me a picture of a well-dressed businessman.

JM: You might want to ask [McTeer] about him. This is fascinating!

Jan: Sheriff McTeer, when did you first become interested in this? [Hoodoo]

McT: On our plantation, we had two witchdoctors, Emiline and Michael. Their grandfathers had been witchdoctors in Africa. They were old, old, when I was a child. And, my grandmother had a high-developed sense of ESP, and my mother inherited it from her. They could foresee things that actually came true. I inherited a little from them, but I was raised right in the atmosphere [of Hoodoo practice]. Then when I became sheriff, I became exposed to witchdoctors.

JM: I know you stated in an earlier interview that you lost around eighty people a year to witchcraft down here [in the Beaufort area], and I was wondering; what could the law do to these people.

McT: Nothing, unless they [the witchdoctors] give them medicine. When I got in a [magical] fight with Dr. Buzzard, he was giving medicine for syphilis, giving medicine for cancer. I told him he had to quit, and when he didn't quit, then he and I went at each other [magically].

JM: Is that what caused the big feud? Telling him he had to quit giving out medicine?

McT: Yeah!

Our conversation was interrupted so that Mr. McTeer could take a telephone call.

Jan: [*to me, referring to another client's letter*] What is this?

JM: This is a lady with a Ph.D., and she feels that her husband is working voodoo on her and he's trying to kill her. She's asking for help.

Jan: [*to McTeer*] What advice would you give this woman?

McT: I'd give her advice on how to protect herself and other things. There's
       a lot more to it [Hoodoo] than just what you see.

JM: I'm sure there is. Let me ask you something. Why aren't there any
       women root doctors?

McT: There are! Oh, yes, indeed! There are plenty of them ... right here
       in Beaufort.... I am the only true white African witchdoctor in
       America, and I'm recognized as being one of the top authorities on
       witchcraft.

The conversation was again interrupted by business, and upon resuming,
turned again to healing practices.

McT: Some of it is psychosomatic ... mind over matter.... Some people
       come in here paralyzed, some insane.... But when they come in,
       I have that much [psychic] ability to know exactly what they are
       thinking, and I know they have come to me b-ecause they know I
       can help them.... They want me to help them.... I've had them be
       carried in here. I've had 'em bring 'em here in the back of Cadillac
       cars by nurses that have been in the family for years, and they can't
       talk and yet the [medical] doctors tell me they can talk but they are
       under a spell.

McT: [to Jan] Would you be interested in seeing where I do all of this?

McTeer was referring to the back room where the magical treatments are
       given.

Jan: I'd love to see it!

McT: Come on back. Do you have a camera?

At this point, we walked through the small hallway to a small back room
that was sparsely decorated, except for a wall hanging comprised of a huge
shell of a horseshoe crab painted to resemble a spirit face. The altar was
covered with various items both natural and commercially manufactured
which McTeer used for magical his work. After viewing the altar room and
work area, we returned to the office.

Jan: Some of these letters are from Hans Holzer [a well-known psychic and author of many such publications in the 1970s]. Does he come here a lot? What association do you have with Hans Holzer?

McT: He's a psychic, and at first, he was a little sarcastic with me, but I put him in his place so damn fast he didn't know how he got there. He and I became friends after that. (McTeer then turned toward me.) How long have you been studying this?

JM: I've been mostly working in the library for a good while. We have also been to visit the Oyotunji Voodoo village located in Shelton. What is your opinion, from what you know and your experience of them?

Oyotunji Village is an African American commune that began in the early 1970s and exists to this day. The founders were attempting to recreate an authentic, Orisha Voodoo-based African community. As Rod Davis says of Oyotunji in his excellent book, *American Voudou: Journey into a Hidden World,* "Oyotunji is not an African village, for Oyotunji is not a place that grew in Africa. It is a place where Africa grows" (182). Although I visited Oyotunji in 1974 as part of my research, I soon realized it had little to do with the traditional world of the Low Country root doctor, so I have not included it in this memoir. I would heartily recommend Davis's book to anyone wishing to know more about this unique community. McTeer's attitudes toward Oyotunji were typical of the Beaufort community in 1974.

McT: My experience is this, that they are opportunists. That he [the self-proclaimed king of the commune] has found an easy way to make a living. He has four or five wives [as of 1975], which is very desirable if the state's supporting you. Everything is free. But, he has a lot of African customs and rituals he's learned, and he's combined that with his sacrifices. He sacrifices goats, chickens and all, and he has a very remunerative thing there by putting black magic on people. I've had people offer me five hundred dollars if I will [use magic to] kill someone's husband with black magic. So, he can make a lot of money. But with me, since I only heal people and won't use witchcraft to kill, anyway, there's no charge whatsoever.

Jan: [*reading an article about Hoodoo*] It says that now it's more prevalent among the whites then the blacks.

JM: What would you attribute that to?

McT: The economy!

JM: The economy?

McT: Sure! I mean, the average man, years ago, started saving his dimes, then he started saving his silver dollars. Putting them away, putting them away.... Why was he doing that? In the back of his mind was the fact that the only basic value was gold and silver. It has happened all through the ages, Civil War and the Revolution too.... It all comes down to insecurity—insecurity and then a lot of people coming into a lot of money that aren't used to it. Like I said about one of my friends—he doesn't know how to wear his money well, you know? He wasn't used to it, so they're seeking, seeking for something. I have gone out with the richest people in the world, even went hunting with [famous New York heiress] Barbara Hutton's father.... He thought I was a good shot ... and they had done everything in the world that could be done. They had power, sex, anything and they had nothing to do. Money had bought him everything that it could buy, and so he just followed the seasons, hunting.

JM: Sort of like the old saying "Lay not your treasures upon the earth." So, this is why the white people come to you, because they have put their treasures upon the earth and left their spirituality out?

McT: That's exactly right!

JM: Have black people kept their spirituality?

McT: The blacks are like everyone else. They have their spirituality when they are in church, but when they get out, they forget it.

Jan: [*still reading from McTeer's correspondence*] Jack, did you know Doctor Snake and Doctor Crow were women?

JM: No, I didn't know that.

McT: They were very powerful, very spiritual women. They could heal and they could kill. Most of the old witchdoctors were like that, the good and the bad were two sides of the same coin.

JM: [*referring to another piece of correspondence*] It says here that many root doctors were located right in this general area.

McT: Sure, Doctor Buzzard was located over on St. Helena Island. Doctor Bug was located on Laurel Bay. Doctor Hawk and Doctor Eagle were located in Beaufort.

JM: I just want to ask, what usually becomes of an old root doctor? You said in one interview that he [Doctor Buzzard] became infatuated with his own power. Does this bring about his destruction?

McT: No, old age, the physical things. He believes in his powers. He's seen so many people get up and walk out after he's treated them, and he's seen so many things happen to people who he put a curse on, he says to himself "I've got the power!" But old age comes for him just the same.

JM: Back in the times before the Civil War, how prevalent was the [Hoodoo] practice?

McT: Before the Civil war was when the slaves came. That was when the true African witchdoctors worked together, and, brother, they were the real bosses on those plantations. Harriet Tubman, you remember her; she ended up here and was decorated here in Beaufort. She led the Underground Railroad right through here. She was a witchdoctor from Africa. Those slaves would do anything Harriet Tubman said, and she could go among them and find out whether Confederate forces were near; she could make the slaves leave with her or strike in the rice fields. She did a lot towards defeating the Confederacy. She got her authority from her heritage as a witchdoctor.

JM: How old are you, Mr. McTeer?

McT: Seventy-one.

JM: Have you ever had someone come to you with a drug problem?

McT: Funny thing, I have never had a drug addict come to me who was under a spell of witchcraft. The two are not connected. Now, I've had mothers beg me: "Get my son off drugs! Someone's put a spell on him to make him take drugs!"

JM: How do these folks know they have a spell on them?

McT: Oh, they feel or sense someone in the house at night. They hear things around the bed; they feel a presence or see something come through the door. When they walk in the yard, they get a burning sensation in their legs 'cause someone has buried a root on them [using contagious magic] a thousand different ways.

JM: I have heard that a root doctor will, if he's heard someone feels the presence of a root, he will sneak in and plant something and let the person find it.

McT: Oh, I did that once, when I treated a lady who wanted to put a curse on me, and it worked. She was in here the next morning to make peace.

JM: I have read that if a white witchdoctor takes money for what he does, that he will lose his ability and the spell won't work.

McT: That's right! If he takes money for helping a person who is in dire trouble, he loses his power. Now, if they want to give him something, he can recommend that they send a contribution to Easter Seals or crippled children or something like that. That's okay!

Jan: Do you ever go to the Oyotunji village?

McT: Yeah, I do. And they come in here with their robes to see me. Yeah, I've been over there many times.

JM: When we were there, it seemed that they were sincere, but they were also very commercial about it also.

McT: Yeah, they're moneymakers and they get everything from the government they can get—free health care, free eyeglasses, free dental care, free baby deliveries.

JM: But they claim they've never gone to the doctor!

McT: Pshaw! The health care truck is over there every week.

JM: But this is not indigenous to Beaufort County.

McT: Not a bit.

JM: I just sensed that there was something. . . .

McT: Synthetic.

JM: Yes, synthetic. I hope you did not mind my calling you the other night.

McT: Not a bit! You're the kind of person I say yes to. . . .

During my interviews with Mr. McTeer, I found a sincere, kind gentleman who was dedicated to helping those who came to him. In several cases we discussed, he guided people away from the practice of Hoodoo as a way of protecting the person from their own foolhardy activities. I believe he enjoyed the attention of our interviews; he certainly did not show outward signs of egotism. He may not have been a sheriff anymore, but he was a shaman who worked his magic for the good of the community. We will not see his level of grace and personal style again.

CHAPTER THREE

Powwowing: Magic in the Piedmont

The Universe is full of magical things, patiently waiting for our wits to grow sharper.

—Eden Philpotts

Love and magic have a great deal in common. They enrich the soul, delight the heart. And they both take practice.

—Nora Roberts

A Little Bit of History

The American shamanic tradition and persona with which I became the most familiar with during my college research and over the past thirty years is known variously as *Powwowing, Braucherei, Using, Using for Sympathy,* or *Hexerei* (in its more spirit-oriented form). I found the terms often used interchangeably, depending on the geographic location of its practitioners. Powwowing is a traditional German American healing art used by skilled practitioners upon humans and animals. It is also a shamanic practice dealing with the world of spirits. In "Powwowing: A Persistent Healing Tradition," published in the *Pennsylvania German Review*, David W. Kriebel defines Powwow as:

> . . . a magico-religious practice whose chief purpose is the healing of physical ailments in humans and animals, although it has had other aims as well, such as conferring protection from physical and spiritual harm, bringing good luck, and revealing hidden information. (17)

In his essay entitled "Braucher's Progress: A Preliminary Reevaluation of Pennsylvania German Folk Medicine," historian Dennis Boyer says of Powwow's origins:

. . . a few sources cited practices derived from Hildegard of Bingen or ascribed to ancient Druids. There are enough tantalizing tidbits suggestive of pre-Christian shamanic practices to merit exploration of the practices of the Germanic tribes and the Celtic tribes they absorbed. (4)

Along with the first German settlers to the new world, Powwow quietly immigrated and blended into the framework of its new environment. Although predominantly Germanic in origin, within one hundred years of the first settlements, elements of Powwow were practiced by a wide variety of ethnic backgrounds including Appalachian, African-American, and Scots-Irish folk healing traditions. Powwow also included elements of 17th-century German Pietism, Cabalistic and Rosicrucian mysticism and American Spiritualism. Powwow borrowed and blended with each of these cultural traditions to become a true American hybrid. Powwow was a name some historians believe was given to the practice by Native Americans who, upon seeing the healing practices, thought that it resembled the actions of their medicine men. This healing practice went by many names and the vocabulary evolved drawing from a variety of cultures. Boyer observed:

> Powwowing adherents came to be marginalized to such an extent that its practitioners might have become increasingly isolated. This may have made them prone to pick up fragments and nonsensical references from other sources and traditions. (10)

Powwow has received little attention in the popular press other than occasional references in novels and movies, such as the Silver Jack series by Appalachian author Manly Wade Wellman, whose protagonist uses Powwow; and the 1987 movie, *Apprentice to Murder,* starring Donald Sutherland, which is loosely based on the 1928 Powwow-related murder of Nelson D. Rehmeyer. Although not following the actual history of this notorious case, the movie gives an accurate picture of Powwowing and the shamanic perceptive mindset that develops as a result of the practice.

The Time and Place: Powwow Emigrates to the Dutch Fork

To begin to understand this complex shamanic practice, it is important to take time to explore the history of how the practice of Powwow came to be in America and eventually into South Carolina's "Dutch Fork" where I found it in 1974.

One must keep in mind that, like the practice of Hoodoo in the Low Country, the geographic boundary for the practice of Powwow is not distinct or confined to a particular area. In this context, we are dealing only with a concentration of a particular shamanic culture. In the examination of Powwow, we are focusing on an area in the middle of South Carolina, locally known as the Piedmont. In the Piedmont, just above the capital city of Columbia, situated roughly between the Broad and Saluda rivers, is an area settled by people primarily from Germany. The word "Dutch" came from a corruption of the word "Deutsch" in German; hence, the "Dutch Fork." The use of the word "Fork" to describe the land between the Broad and Saluda rivers was employed in land warrants as early as 1744, and the phrase "Dutch Fork between Saluda and Broad Rivers" appears in a 1794 Act of the General Assembly of South Carolina. The Dutch Fork area was referred to early in its settlement as Saxe-Gotha, as we will see from historical documents noted below.

This geographically beautiful area of South Carolina called the Piedmont is still characterized by a mixture of small towns and farms nestled in the gently rolling hills. The terrain is a deep red clay soil with a predominance of hardwood trees, unlike the pine forests of the Low Country. The Piedmont was decidedly rural until the early 1960s, when it was discovered by land developers searching for places to expand Columbia's rapidly growing population. In a short, 30-year period, the area evolved from a rural to a suburban community, with all that such a transformation entails.

My family moved there in 1965 in an early phase of this expansion, so I was still able to enjoy the many advantages of living in what our former friends from Columbia called "the sticks." As a result, I spent countless hours wandering the woods; exploring old abandoned farmhouses and moonshine stills and watching the freight trains speed by. It is hard to imagine now, driving in some areas of the St. Andrews' section with its modern suburban sprawl, how it once appeared. One can still get a glimpse of the old Dutch Fork, however, by driving up the Old Newberry Highway or some other quiet back road. The once small town of Lexington, South Carolina, where

I met with my primary Powwow contact, Lee Raus Gandee, has grown to the point that I can no longer find my way to his former residence. It was in the Dutch Fork that the practice of Powwow was concentrated, so let us now examine its unique cultural history.

It is worth remembering that two of the factors that led to the colonization of America by European settlers came under the broad categories of necessity and inclination, not the least of which were due to political and religious persecution. Every schoolchild knows about the Puritans, who arrived on the barren rocks and shores of Plymouth, Massachusetts. Later, the Carolinas saw the arrival of the Huguenots of France, the Nonconformists of Scotland, the German Palatines (Pfalzer) from the Rhine, and the Salzburgers from the Alpine districts of Austria. They were seeking neither wealth nor fortune, simply the freedom to worship the Divine in their own ways.

G. D. Bernheim, in his book *History of the German Settlements and of the Lutheran Church in North and South Carolina*, published in 1872, wrote:

> These noble colonists erected many a Plymouth monument of religious liberty on our Southern shores, and under circumstances much more interesting than those which attended the crossing of the noted Mayflower from Old to New England. (133)

The Settlement

From the outset, life was both difficult and dangerous for the new settlers.

In *History of St. Andrews and the Dutch Fork,* historian Daniel W. Hollis wrote:

> After the colony of South Carolina had narrowly escaped disaster in the Yemassee War and Pirate Crisis of 1715-1719, Governor Robert Johnson, acutely aware of the menace of "external and internal enemies" (excessively large Negro slave population and Indians), designed a plan to entice "foreign Protestant" settlers to South Carolina. In about 1730 nine townships, located in the central area of South Carolina, were set up ... into which a steady influx of German settlers began to pour in the 1730's. (5-6)

When good land in Saxe-Gotha became scarce, Hollis noted, "enterprising settlers pushed across the 'Saludy' River into the Fork" (5-6). There is some indication, however, that the first settlers in the Fork may have been English or Scots-Irish pioneers who came in from the Broad River side. According to Hollis,

> The first "Dutch" or German settlers in the Fork were German Swiss, many of which came to South Carolina in the 1740's, but the influx of Swiss Germans stopped in about 1748 as a result of Swiss laws prohibiting immigration. After about 1750 the Dutch Fork settlers came from Baden and Wurtenburg, German provinces on the Rhine River adjacent to Switzerland. Having endured decades of brutal warfare, the tyranny of petty princes, and religious persecution, the Rhinelanders were attracted by the offer of land and the prospect of a new home that would be free of their current harassments. . . . As of 1760 some 2,000 Germans had settled in the Fork, pushing up to Cannons Creek on the Broad and to Beaver Dam Creek on the Saluda. The German influx dropped off sharply in the 1760s. As of 1765 the German and Scotch-Irish newcomers had received scant attention from the provincial government in Charles Town. (5-6)

A decided lack of attention by the colonial government marked the early history of the Dutch Fork area, which formed the character and social atmosphere of the settlers. The area was plagued with needs that were almost never met, the most urgent of which were: law enforcement, courts, political representation, educational facilities, medical attention and structured religious guidance.

To illustrate the problems the early settlers and their descendants faced, the circumstances surrounding the needs above are supported by relevant historical documentation, when such records could be located.

Law Enforcement

> The almost complete lack of law enforcement led to the outbreak of a major crime wave in the aftermath of the Cherokee War. Few of the lawbreakers were natives of the Fork, but in 1767 an outlaw gang cut a wide swath through the area stealing horses, robbing and burning houses and barns. In the absence of sheriffs and constables the outraged up country-men formed a vigilante organization known as the Regulators and put down the crime wave. (Hollis 6)

According to Bernheim,

> One evening in the year 18—, I cannot now recall the exact date, a man
> named Thompson, who lived about four miles from the Court House
> (Newberry, S. C.), came into the village and told the people that there
> were five hundred Negro men collected together, just above where Jalapa
> now stands, for the purpose of burning the village and killing everybody
> in it. There was great excitement; the women went into the hotel and
> into the Court House to be guarded. Every man in the village who had a
> gun was making all the haste he could for a fight. Sentinels were stationed
> all around the village. (501)

Courts

As Hollis noted, "Among the most urgent needs of the up country were
law enforcement and courts" (6).

The fact that the principals involved in the atrocities of the "Weberite
Heresy" had to be taken to trial in Charles Town, 130 miles from the Dutch
Fork, implies that courts were not available in the Saxe-Gotha area at that
time. The Weberite Heresy was an early American case of a destructive
religious cult, not unlike those tragic groups that have made headlines in
recent decades, such as the Peoples Temple in Jonestown, Guyana, and the
Branch Davidians in Waco, Texas.

This earlier cult, which centered in and around the town of Little
Mountain, South Carolina, had as its focus, a charismatic individual named
Jacob Weber, who began to have religious meetings in his home somewhere
around 1761. A few key people were singled out by Weber, as he became
more involved in what he perceived as his mission—with disastrous consequences. According to Brenda Reed's reprint of the writings of Lutheran
church leader Rev. Henry Melchior Muhlenberg's account of the Weberite
Heresy, Weber and his wife Hannah, began receiving what they interpreted
to be mystical revelations. Apparently, Weber then

> proclaimed himself to be God and Hannah "the Virgin Mary"; Johann
> Georg Schmidtpeter or John George Smithpeter, the "Son of God"; "a
> godless colored preacher named Dauber," the Holy Spirit. (Muhlenberg
> qtd. in Reed, par. 1)

As the cult grew and new members were attracted, the four principals began quarreling over doctrine and power. Before the militia was eventually summoned from Charleston, the cult had wreaked havoc on the little community and murdered at least three men, one by trampling him to death under a mattress.

Once order was restored, the principals were taken to Charleston and eventually Jacob Weber was hanged. It was a tragic chapter in the history of the backcountry and a lesson on following charismatic religious leaders that has been lost on future generations. Among the circumstances that contributed to the development of such a cult was the physical isolation of the backcountry and lack of formal religious leadership. This is evidenced by a passage from Rev. Muhlenberg, in Bernheim:

> But in the rural districts of South Carolina, the spiritual condition of the German settlers was most deplorable, inasmuch as, previous to the year 1737, not a single German pastor labored among them. The Lutherans in Saxe-Gotha Township, numbering two hundred and eighty souls, wrote to the Ebenezer pastors, in 1750, for a minister of their own faith; but their urgent plea was not regarded, which greatly discouraged them. Need anyone be astonished at the legitimate effects of so deplorable a want of the means of grace as was witnessed at that time in the Province of South Carolina. (Muhlenberg qtd. in Bernheim 196-197)

Political Representation

> "The up countrymen were virtually unrepresented in the General Assembly, the tax laws were grossly unfair, the capital was located at distant Charles Town" (Hollis 6).

Bernheim reflected on the lack of consideration for the feeling of the upcountry German communities in the General Assembly:

> Saxe-Gotha comprised of nearly all that portion of territory embraced at present in Lexington County; it is not many years since the name was changed, in honor of the battle of Lexington, Massachusetts, by an act of legislature, which was a most unfortunate exchange of names, being less euphonic, very inappropriate, and altogether unhistorical. Give us back the old name, and may the citizens of old Saxe-Gotha, in South Carolina, never be ashamed of their German extraction. (196)

This sense of cultural disenfranchisement carried over into a general lack of interest in the concerns of the colony in the coast that carried over to the American Revolution:

> The grievance of the Germans against the Charles Town leaders who favored the Revolution was far greater than the resentment against a king who had given them land and who had permitted far more political, economic, and religious freedom than they had known in Germany. The Sugar Act, Stamp Act, Declaratory Act, the Boston Massacre and Boston Tea Party meant little to the isolated Forkers. Consequently, when young William Henry Drayton came from Charles Town in 1755 to rally backcountry support for the Revolutionary cause he received a cold reception. Failing to secure a single adherent in the Dutch Fork, the patriotic firebrand was happy to leave such a "stiff-necked generation." (Hollis 7)

Hollis further notes, "The fact that the South Carolina 'Dutch' have tended to forego politics may be partially responsible for the neglect they have received from Palmetto writers" (11).

During the American Revolution, Hessian mercenaries came upon settlers of German descent, who still spoke their native language. According to Bernheim, the mercenaries "deserted the ranks of the British army whenever they found a safe opportunity" (174) and were welcomed into the Saxe-Gotha community, later known as the Dutch Fork.

Educational Facilities

> But it is possible that, as in the State of New York, the benevolent Queen Anne did make grants of land for church and school purposes in Saxe-Gotha Township, which, however, could not be occupied at the time, as the settlements in South Carolina had then not been extended so far inland; the Indians were still in possession of that portion of the province, and the grants and good intentions of the Queen were eventually lost sight of and forgotten. (Bernheim 128)

An additional characteristic of the Germans who settled the Dutch Fork was that they did not culturally disperse and assimilate into the new American society, as did other settlers, but remained together as a cultural group, staunchly devoted to their Lutheranism and their language. These settlers also tended to marry within the community.

Medical Attention

John Hawkins, in his 1907 article for *Popular Science Monthly*, "Magical Medical Practice in South Carolina," noted,

> Until ninety or a hundred years ago, according to local historians, there were no physicians in this region. Besides the stock of medical lore in the possession of the old women of every country neighborhood, the sick had recourse only to a system of practice known as "using. . . ." (166)

John Belton O'Neall, in his book, *The Annals of Newberry*, noted, "The people in Dutch Fork had no doctors in those happy days. All diseases were cured by our Dutch doctors by *using*—all being done in German" (482).

Despite their social isolation and numerous deprivations, as the years rolled by, these hearty settlers managed to forge communities that were law-abiding, productive and independent. The people of the area were known for their honesty, generosity and hospitality. O'Neall included Colonial Army Major J. P. Kinard's statement: "Never were there more honest and just people on the face of the earth than Germans in those days" (481).

Powwow Survives as a Cultural Legacy

By now, the reader will have reached the conclusion that the early settlers of the Dutch Fork region addressed themselves to their own needs and problems as best they could. They managed, for better or worse, and strengthened their cultural insularity. This insularity gave Powwow fertile ground to survive, develop and grow unseen and unmolested by the outer world.

People of the German settlements of South Carolina still held to their traditional beliefs in healing and traced these beliefs to their pre-Christian origins. According to Hawkins,

> In old Germany neither Charlemagne's conquest nor the priest that followed it could put a period to the use of staves carved with mystic runes and devoted to the purposes of divination and incantation. The oak, the ash, and the willow preserved their sacred character; and in the old heathen

formulas used for the cure of disease, the only change effected by Christianity was the substitution of the three highest names (Father, Son and Holy Ghost) for those of Thor, Woden and other heathen deities. (170)

Some fifty-odd years later, Hexenmeister Lee Raus Gandee, in his article, "'Using' to Heal in South Carolina," published in *Fate Magazine* in 1961, wrote,

It is not difficult to find "users" today and they "use" for many purposes. Almost every community in the Dutch Fork and the surrounding German area has some man or woman who can "use to stop blood," and "use to draw fire" There have been famous "users" who were conceded to have the power to cure goiter, diseases of the throat, of the eyes, even cancer. (35)

Are these references sufficient for us to conclude that the Powwow system has indeed transcended the years from colonial days to the present in the Dutch Fork? It is important to remember that Powwow practitioners, along with historians and researchers in modern times, are still the carriers of the tradition and its history.

Powwow did not only develop in South Carolina but became part of the American landscape wherever Germans settled. Until this point in the narrative, I have emphasized the history and presence of Powwow in South Carolina, with concentration on the Dutch Fork region. I would be remiss by not covering, to some degree, another center of the Powwow tradition in North America, which is spiritually and culturally connected to the early Dutch Fork community.

Other Famous Powwows of the Dutch Fork:
Granny Slice, Daniel Koon and Aunt Tiny

Granny Slice

In his book, *Strange Experience: Secrets of a Hexenmeister,* Lee Gandee relates the unusual story of "Old Granny Slice, the good witch of Dutch Fork, [who] would start across a blazing woodland, and how people marveled when the fire died at her tracks."

No one I had interviewed had actually seen Granny Slice perform her "fire walking"—after all she had been dead for a number of years. By the mid-1970s, however, she and her ability had become the stuff of local legend. No one knew of anyone who could perform such a feat anymore, and with the exception of Lee, most seemed uncomfortable talking about such things.

Granny Slice's fire-walking and the healing of animals especially appeared to challenge the notion that the success of sympathetic healing is based on the awareness and faith of the person receiving the treatment.

Lil' Daniel Koon

There were other Powwows in the Dutch Fork area that were famous for their abilities, including the traditional art of shape-shifting. Lee often spoke of a farmer named Daniel Koon (1810–1876), who resided in the area near Chapin, South Carolina.

On the website of the Palmetto Genealogy Association, "Believe it or Not: South Carolina Folklore" (*www.palmettoroots.org/SCFolklore.html*), Marlene Koon Walker, going through Koon family papers, offers the following insights into the personality and magical practices of Daniel Koon:

> According to John Belton O'Neall in *The Annals of Newberry* "many among the Germans once believed in using, that is the cure of disease by catalistic words, and passing the hand of the operator over the part of the body or limb affected. . . . Since mesmerism has become fashionable, and is believed by many intelligent, well-educated men, I confess I cannot see why using should not also be. It is but another name for mesmerism . . . if a college of instruction in mesmerism was to be established in this State, I think Dr. Coon has more claims to be President than any man within my knowledge. (par. 1)

> Lee Gandee, in a letter to Carl W. Nichols of Aug. 30, 1972, relates of a conversation with a Mr. Linda in which he is informed "Daniel Coon was the greatest user that ever was in the Fork" . . . and then he told me of the times that "Lei's Dan's" used to make himself invisible and let people get them scared senseless by walking by them and talking, or of making them see him as a fence post, or as a log or stump and then letting them see him appear in his own form. (par. 2)

Even the old history of Newberry mentions "Dr. Koon" (Daniel), saying in connection with the rage for Mesmerism that involved the Summer, Meyer, and Chapman families in the 1850s, that if Mesmerism could be a socially acceptable matter, so could "using" and that Dr. Koon could probably show any Mesmerist a few things that the latter could not equal. I was exceeding lucky to pick up the books on Mesmerism that Summer got for Mrs. Chapman, and given a while to prepare the girls and Mrs. Wessinger in advance, by means of it I also could make them see a head with a long beard, on the ground by the spring, in place of mine, and not see the body at all. The Koons were fabulous Mesmerists (Hypnotists), and genuine practitioners of magic. Daniel and seven grimoires that his children would not even touch, and he could read German, Latin, French, Hebrew and English and create spells with them all. (par. 4)

Coy Bayne, in *Lake Murray: Legend and Leisure*, provides additional insights into Daniel Koon's everyday personality (from the website "Believe it or Not: South Carolina Folklore"):

The Dutch Germans who settled "in the fork" were often intelligent, well-read and hardworking. One example was Daniel Koon of the Chapin area who was born in 1810 and died in 1876. (par. 1)

Daniel was well read and had a library of books. He taught children to fear his books in order to protect them from handling. He could speak four languages. (par. 2)

He was also an expert craftsman and wheelwright, but his greatest reputation lay in his strange talents of being able to stop bleeding, soothing burns, curing thrash and talking children into deep, restful sleep. He admitted to being a "faith healer" but insisted he was no doctor nor did he pretend to have any special powers. Nevertheless, when neighbors sent for him night or day he hurried to them. He said he could soothe the ill by reassurance. He never refused sharing his talents nor did he ever charge for his services. (par. 3)

He had a widespread reputation for mystery and may have contributed to this image by clever manipulation. When Sherman troop's came to the Koon house at the end of the Civil War, they went to his barn to take his two mules and a horse. As they opened the gate, the animals burst free, knocking the soldiers out of the way and disappearing into the woods. The soldiers ransacked Koon's smokehouse and when his dog's began growling at them the soldiers shot at the dogs. They missed each time and the dogs escaped. Koon went to a wash pot, reached down into it and came up with a handful of pistol balls. He told the soldiers their bullets had gone to the wash pot. The frustrated soldiers hurriedly grouped and departed promptly taking no other belongings. The horse and mules came home two weeks later. (par. 4)

Other families also have stories of relatives who practiced powwow at a very high level. Vickie Ellisor, writes about "Aunt Tiny" on the "Believe it or Not: South Carolina Folklore, in "More Interesting Tales: 'Was She a Witch or Not?'"

My grandmother told me one night that her Aunt Tiny, was a witch and that she could turn herself into any animal except a dove and a lamb. She said that her father went to catch a 'possum for Sunday's lunch and Aunt Tiny liked to play tricks on the men folk. She turned herself into a fat 'possum and let them catch her. The men captured her and placed her (Aunt Tiny) in a crocker sack. They threw the sack on the porch and went in to grab a quick bite to eat. My grandmother's father said, "I better go and get the 'possum before Tiny get a hold of it." When he reached for the bag, he found it empty! Aunt Tiny had turned herself into a horse and was standing at the kitchen door with her head in the kitchen (it was one of those pleat-doors) and was laughing. My grandmother's father came in to the kitchen and said, "Where is Tiny? The 'possum is gone." When he had finished saying that Tiny had turned herself back to her own self and my grandmother's father had to go out and find something else for them to eat for lunch on Sunday. (par. 1)

As you can imagine, these are people who lived within the then small, rural communities of the Dutch Fork and practiced a form of shamanism and Powwow. If there are still such people, I have not heard of them. One reason may be the social incursions due to demographic changes in the St. Andrews, Lake Murray and greater Columbia metropolitan communities. These changes have brought unparalleled growth to the area in population, housing and community development. "The old Lexington is gone!" a clerk in a convenience store remarked to me last year as I tried, without success, to locate Lee Gandee's former home. "Everything has just grown by leaps and bounds. There's not much left the way it used to be."

The Pennsylvania Historical Connection

Another cultural center for the Powwow tradition is located in Pennsylvania, and may have begun in the area known as Germantown near Philadelphia. Originally established as a religious colony along the Wissahickon Creek, the settlers were a group called the Brothers of the Society of the Woman in the Wilderness. Firmly believing that the end of time was near, this community of Pietists, under the leadership of Magister Johannes Kelpius, came to Pennsylvania in 1694. They, along with other groups, crossed the Atlantic Ocean to enjoy the promise of religious freedom provided by Pennsylvania's Quaker-based legal system. Their history is chronicled by historian Julius Friedrich Sachse, former president of the Pennsylvania–German Society, in his book, *The German Pietists of Provincial Pennsylvania 1694-1708*. This group's unusual name referred to a character, who "mentioned in Revelation xii, 14-17, was prefigurative of the great deliverance that was then soon to be displayed for the Church of Christ" (Sachse 80). The Pietists were a group of European Christian mystics who sought spiritual perfection in Gnosis and in Divine revelation. Sachse said they "were also a true Theosophical (Rosicrucian) Community, a branch of that ancient mystical brotherhood who studied and practiced the Kabbala" (62).

The German Pietists were referred to as "Sect People," who desired to avoid war and religious persecution. They had embarked from London aboard the *Sarah Maria* on February 13, 1694, bound for Pennsylvania. After a rigorous voyage, they finally landed at Philadelphia on Saturday, June 24, 1694. During the months that followed, they established a reclusive community on the banks of the Wissahickon, and subsequently, the Cocalico River, in an area known as Hermits Glen. They resided in this area in separate caves along the hillside, where they practiced their rituals and beliefs unmolested for several decades, until the American Revolution. Subsequent immigration began to eat away at their seclusion, and as the principals died off, the younger generations moved away, joining, in many cases, secularized churches. While the history of these people is interesting, the beliefs and customs they brought with them to this country made their reclusive existence somewhat legendary and the extent of their influence cannot be measured. Sachse noted their generosity: "All services of a spiritual, educational and medical nature were given free, without price or hope of fee or reward" (83).

The Pietists believed that they could not only spiritually but also physically regenerate their existence in order to achieve perfection. Sachse describes their spiritual goal:

> The great object of these speculations was to reach the nearest approach that man can make to the unseen, that inner companion which works silently in the soul, but which cannot be expressed in absolute language, nor by any words, which is beyond all formulations into word-symbolism, yet is on the confines of the unknown spiritual world. This state, it was held, could only be obtained away from the allurements of the world by entering into silence, meditation and inner communion with one's self. With the absolute negation of all world matter, thought and world-matter existence, or in other words, the nearest approach to the Invisible can only be reached by the acknowledgement of the Non-Ego. (64)

In addition to this brief introduction to their philosophy, these mystics, upon arrival in Philadelphia, celebrated the pre-Christian rites of *Sommeuriend fleur*, or St. John's Eve, on June 24 and December 25. This ceremony celebrates the recurrence of the summer and winter solstices for the purpose of allaying any possible pestilence and disease. The embers of the large bonfire of flowers, pine boughs and bones were then cast over the surrounding area.

A Digression: The Past Meets Contemporary Times in the Dutch Fork

I must interrupt our early historical journey at this point to indicate that these same rites were carried out in the Dutch Fork in rural Lexington County in 1970, according to Lee Gandee, in a field off Route 7. I make note of this contemporary event to alert readers to three further points I wish to make, which will explain why I have related certain details in the history of an obscure group of mystics in Pennsylvania.

First, Sachse's book *The German Pietists of Provincial Pennsylvania, 1694–
1708,* was published in 1895, and only 500 copies were printed. Yet, Lee
Gandee's copy, numbered 429, was in the Dutch Fork within one year of its
publication. It is signed by the author and his son, and carries an inscription
indicating it was a gift to a Dutch Fork resident, Ralph Entriker. Its boards
and pages were festooned with Powwow symbols, which were meticulously
drawn and painted by hand. It also included inscriptions in German to
protect the contents of the book and the home in which it resided from
theft, destruction or harm.

Second, the sect of German Pietists noted above was known throughout
Germantown and all of Eastern Pennsylvania for their amazing and often
magical deeds and kind acts. It is important to mention here that they were
known by the term "Hexenmeister." Two of the most famous Hexenmeisters
in the contemporary history of Hexerei were Christopher Witt and Conrad
Matthai, whose acts are not only legendary but, in some cases, according to
Sachse, are documented historically.

Conrad Matthai was the last official leader of the Wissahickon community. By all accounts, he was a gentle, humble and pious hermit who
dressed in homespun clothes, had long hair and a beard and carried a long
traditional German walking staff. Matthai was best known for his shaman-
like psychic abilities and "was respected by the aged and reputable citizens,
feared by the frivolous and by children and the superstitiously inclined . . .
was avoided as a supernatural being" (Sachse 390). Once, at the request of
the concerned wife of a sea captain who traveled from the coast to find
him, Matthai lay down upon the board upon which he slept and passed
into a deep trance, causing the woman a one point to think he was dead.
After some time, he emerged from the trance. Matthai told the worried
woman that her husband was safe. He said that during his trance, he had
met with her husband in a London coffeehouse, relayed her concerns and
reported that her husband had been delayed and would return soon. When
the husband arrived home as predicted, the curious wife asked her husband
to travel with her to meet Matthai. According to Sachse, upon spotting the
old man, the captain

... told his wife that he has seen this very man upon such a day (it was the day that the woman had made her visit) in a coffeehouse in London and that he [Matthai] came to him telling him how distressed was his wife that he had not written. (394)

We will see that Conrad Matthai played a more modern role in my time with Lee Gandee in Chapter 8.

Third, Sachse notes that such men were also present from the southern regions of the United States: "One George Neisser arrived in Pennsylvania in February of 1737 from Georgia to join the community that was being founded" (6). This well-known trail north from Georgia to Pennsylvania would have passed through South Carolina and the German settlers who would have welcomed Neisser and provided him with a source of food and logistical support. The community was well known enough to be included in the writings of Rev. Henry Melchior Muhlenberg, who praised the community for its acts of personal kindness and spiritual instruction to Lutherans living in the Germantown area. You may recall that Muhlenberg also wrote the account of the Weberites mentioned earlier in this chapter.

In short, it is now evident that from the early 1700s, in German settlements, the practice of Powwow and the existence of Hexenmeisters were found in Pennsylvania and in the provincial Carolinas (which at that time included portions of Georgia), but also that these communities were aware of and in contact with each other. There is no reason to suppose that they weren't also sharing their spiritual and magical traditions. The practice of Powwow was one of great sophistication and still in full swing. The resemblance of doctrines and practices was painstakingly covered in Sachse's book, and similarities were found in the practices throughout the Dutch Fork.

In his 1960 book, *Black Rock*, George Korson discusses Powwowing in the mining area of Southern Pennsylvania where, at the time, it

... is still largely practiced about the mines. But when it is remembered that these healers of burns are practical nurses, and experienced in the treatment and bandaging of the injured parts before they recite the charm or incantation the cures they effect are not so remarkable.... When a man was burned at the mines she would attend the case as well as any physician. It was this ability that cured or helped the man and not her powwowing to "draw out the fire." But you could not convince believers in the occult of this. (268)

David Kriebel, in "Powwowing: A Persistent Healing Tradition," points out that in many areas Powwows were held in high personal and spiritual esteem, even to the extent that "some powwowers also came to be viewed as saints" (19). Many of them, like the famous Powwow, "Mountain Mary," were regarded as angels of mercy where there was little other help to be found. Folklorist Barbara Reimensnyder, in *Powwowing in Union County: A Study of Pennsylvania German Folk Medicine in Context,* notes:

> Externally awarded qualifications, such as degrees, licenses, carry less weight in this system than in the scientific point of view. Community approval and a record of successful cures—as well as the authority of the Bible and Christianity . . . justify faith in a particular healer. (44)

It is worth noting that that in all societies that maintain shamans or healers, a successful cure not only restores the physical and spiritual balance of the individual but also restores the social fabric and spiritual balance of the community. Their group-concept of reality has been healed as well.

The Church and the Powwow: An Uneasy Truce

Largely hidden from the prying eyes of society, most traditional and modern practitioners of Powwow would deny any involvement with the paranormal or occult, nor would they recognize the non-Christian roots of their activities. Many of the older Powwows characterize themselves as devout Christians who profess to simply act as vehicles though which God can move and intervene in human affairs. These Powwows consider their ability a special gift of God and therefore never accept compensation for their services.

My Powwow contact in the Dutch Fork, Lee Raus Gandee, wrote in his 1961 *Fate Magazine* article, "'Using' to Heal in South Carolina":

> Healers claimed that their acts were beneficial, that using magic to heal did not constitute sin since the people supported them; the churches made no great attempt to suppress the use of incantations and rituals of healing. (34)

Kriebel, interviewing a traditional, deeply religious female Powwow called Daisy, noted: "Even a U.C.C. [United Church of Christ] minister comes [for treatment] . . . though not the minister of her church" (15).

I do not wish to give the impression that there is wholesale acceptance of these practices by the local religious establishment. On the contrary, many see this as a form of witchcraft or at least outside the proper code of conduct for the church-going faithful, and deem any cures, no matter how effective, to be of a dubious source. According to Jacob J. Hershberger, in John Andrew Hostetler's *Amish Roots: A Treasury of History, Wisdom and Lore*, "He [God] has instructed in his Word for the curing and healing the sick . . . but nowhere has God commanded to perform some of the shenanigans some powwowers have thought up" (107).

On the other hand, however, just as many feel a variety of healing approaches are appropriate. According to Effie Troyer in Hostetler's *Amish Roots*, "We need both the MDs and the chiropractors and yes, those who brauch too" (107).

The traditional practice of not accepting money reflects the Divine source of power and the Powwow's role as transmitter of that energy. Reimensnyder, in her book *Powwowing in Union County: A Study of Pennsylvania German Folk Medicine in Context* records a Pennsylvania Powwow as saying, "But it's the Lord that heals. I couldn't do it. . . . You have to have faith that it's going to help them, [but] it's the Lord that heals" (1).

Finally, Mildred Jordan, in *The Distelfink Country of the Pennsylvania Dutch,* said,

> Many practitioners are serious, usually loyal church members. They deny that powwowing conflicts with medical attention, they've even treated doctors, they claim. One Powwower is a lay medical man who had a license from the Commonwealth of Pennsylvania for nineteen years to manufacture and sell medicine. Most Powwowers claim that no special talent is needed. Didn't Jesus say "what I can do you can do?" (151)

The point remains that Powwow, like other forms of magically based healing, however lauded or criticized, remains outside the established boundaries of conventional society. Yet it also continues to be, to many, another method of seeking relief form some sort of illness or problem.

The Powwow then, with nothing more than hands, herbs and chants, and with roots going back hundreds of years, begins, traveling alongside more conventional healing methods and medicine. Each of us supports the Powwow's work. Why? Because each of us, wittingly or unwittingly, is a keeper of the faith in the spiritual, the magical and the miraculous! As John Wesley, the 18th-century founder of Methodism, is quoted as saying, "Giving up witchcraft is, in effect, giving up the Bible" (Jordan 148).

The Darker Side of Powwow

Powwow, like any other spiritual practice, can have a darker, negative side. This dark side of Powwow was illustrated in the 1987 movie *Apprentice to Murder,* which loosely follows the book *Hex*, written in 1969 by Arthur H. Lewis. *Hex* recounts a murder committed on November 28, 1928, in North Hopewell Township, near York, Pennsylvania, that had Powwowing as a motive. A farmer and Powwow, Nelson D. Rehmeyer, was beaten and murdered by three men who believed he had cursed them. Others have said that Mr. Rehmeyer may have been a professional magical rival to defendant John H. Blymer, who was also known to practice Powwow.

Mr. Rehmeyer's death resulted from the failed attempt of the three men to get a lock of his hair and his copy of *The Long Lost Friend*, a well-known book of ritual-based healing techniques. The three men believed that by stealing Rehmeyer's hair and spell-book, they could break Rehmeyer's curse by burying his hair and book in the earth.

The three accused in the Rehmeyer murder were arrested, tried, convicted and served long prison sentences. In the article "The Witch Murder Verdicts," published in *Literary Digest,* upon hearing his sentence pronounced, defendant John H. Blymer is quoted as saying, "Oh, well, I don't care. The hex Rehmeyer put on me has been gone since his death, and I can eat and sleep now. Even in prison that will be better than it was before" (11).

The sensational coverage of the murder and trial in the national press revealed the practice of Powwow to the modern world. Such publicity caused a good deal of embarrassment to the more educated, urban population, as well as the state officials of Pennsylvania, who, before this incident, seemed to care little about the welfare of these rural folk. The state officials launched a publicity campaign to denounce such superstitions as Powwow and Hex with educational campaigns in the public schools.

According to folklorist Yvonne Milspaw in her 1978 article, "Witchcraft Belief in a Pennsylvania German Family," by the early 1930s, it was announced that, "Public opinion and education had officially banished witchcraft from Pennsylvania" (14). In the 1970s, however, Milspaw discovered that such beliefs had simply gone underground and were still being maintained within families.

As a side note, *The Long Lost Friend* is often found wherever Powwow is practiced and is referred to frequently in this book. It was written in 1820 by Johann Georg (John George) Hohman, and printed in Berks County, Pennsylvania. During the course of my fieldwork, I saw copies in several homes I visited in the Dutch Fork, shelved near the family Bible.

It is worth noting that during my talks with Hexenmeister Lee Gandee, he revealed to me that a somewhat similar incident had occurred in the Dutch Fork during the early 1960s. If Lee's account is to be taken at face value, the story surrounded a Powwow who had begun to practice harmful magic and had become a nuisance to his family and the community. After repeated attempts to reason with him, and with the cooperation of his family, he was forced to flee the community, never to return.

In this section, I have tried to introduce the reader to the historical roots of Powwow and Hexerei practices in America. I have also tried to emphasize that this deeply rooted ancient and mystical belief system is still alive and functioning in most places where Germans who came to America settled; areas such as: Pennsylvania, West Virginia, Ohio, North and South Carolina. I would now like to turn our focus to my main contact during those early days of my research, Lee Raus Gandee.

CHAPTER FOUR

Lee Gandee: Hexenmeister, Teacher, Friend

Reality is nothing but a collective hunch.   —Lilly Tomlin, (1939–)

That so few now dare to be eccentric, marks the chief danger of the time.
     —John Stuart Mill, (1806–1873)

"HOW DOES ONE BECOME a Hexenmeister?" I asked him at our first meeting.

"By being a Hex until you can manage it!" replied the elderly gentleman in the rocking chair, calmly smoking his pipe. This was Lee Raus Gandee, the "Hexenmeister of the Dutch Fork"—and my primary contact into this invisible community. This was the question and answer that began our four-year relationship from 1974 to 1977. Lee Gandee opened my eyes to a world apart, a world beyond any I'd known before and one in which I still find an ever-deepening sense of wonder.

Lee had moved to Lexington County in central South Carolina in the 1940s. He learned Powwow from his maternal grandmother in West Virginia, who had adopted him from his young, troubled mother soon after his birth.

He was a retired history professor, author and hereditary Powwow. Lee Gandee was also a man with a checkered, if not fearsome reputation, in the then-rural community of Lexington, for a variety of reasons that will be explained later.

The year was 1974, and January already felt like spring as I first sat in Lee's rural home with his spacious, combination study and bedroom. He was proud of the fact that he had purchased a true "Hex house." He had recognized that it as a Hex house because it was situated on the highest point of land between two bodies of flowing water and faced west. The house was surrounded by the same oaks and holly trees that its first owner had gazed upon nearly 200 years earlier. The first owner was a woman named Mary Ingelman, who was reputed to be a Powwow and healer. In 1792, in Fairfield County, South Carolina, during an act of mob hysteria, she was tried, convicted and tortured for the crime of witchcraft, long after the infamous Salem witch trials.

As he lived only about fifteen miles from my family home near Irmo, South Carolina, Lee was the most geographically accessible of my field contacts during the early years of my research. I found Lee and Powwow intriguing, as both provided insights into my own German-American heritage, which, I discovered in 1975, included the practice of Powwow by my own maternal great-grandfather. What started as a scholastic pursuit soon became increasingly personal and began to consume my thoughts, time, and energy. It drew me away from the objective, detached posture of a field researcher and into the relationship of pupil to Gandee's role of teacher. In those days, I wrestled with myself on a near-constant basis regarding the proper stance I should take toward what I was experiencing. I tried to deny the fact that I was plunging headlong into it, as the many experiences I had slowly wore down my skepticism.

I suppose I was lucky that I encountered Lee at a time of enormous personal upheaval in his life. It was a period of great personal change, including divorce and deeply strained relationships within his immediate family. This alienation of family combined with Lee's emerging female identity allowed him to rationalize his teaching me, because Powwowing was a traditionally taught cross-gender. I also now believe he felt he would have few opportunities in the future to pass on his tradition. I would also like to think he saw me as a sincere, if not naïve, person with an aptitude and willingness for learning to Powwow.

When I would become frustrated with myself, Lee would become fatherly and remind me to be patient by counseling, "You cannot rush your relationship with this anymore than you can a romantic one, or one with God. You can't hurry the seasons, the rain or anything else in nature.... They all move in their own good time, and you'd better learn to move with them or you will lose yourself for no reason."

As we continued our interviews, I realized that Lee was not only highly educated and well versed in the local history, but he had written a spiritual autobiography entitled *Strange Experience: Autobiography of a Hexenmeister*. In 2002, Hexenmeister Karl Herr, in his book *Hex and Spellwork: The Magical Practices of the Pennsylvania Dutch* noted, "the best of the books about Hexenmeisters is probably Lee R. Gandee's *Strange Experience*" (23).

Lee offered me a copy of *Strange Experience* at the end of our first visit, with the admonishment to read it and "decide whether you really want to come back." Now long out of print, I took it home and pored over it. This account presented itself as one of folklore, magic and intrigue, and included many of his personal and spiritual revelations. I soon realized why he wanted me to know about him as a person before returning to see him again. Immersed in this story of the magical and marvelous was the story of Lee's long struggle with his sexual identity and his emergence as a gay person. Now I understood some of the peculiar questions and reactions I had received from some of the local folks when I initially sought him out. I thought carefully and realized that I was not concerned or bothered by the revelation that Lee was gay, or even that he had a name for his feminine side. What really intrigued me were the stories of Powwow and Hexerei—healing and magic—things beyond the ordinary realm of human experience. I remember thinking to myself, "If this guy is for real, is not crazy and doesn't try to make a pass at me, this could be a great adventure!"

I returned to his house bearing gifts of pipe tobacco and other small items to compensate him for his time, although it soon became clear he would have talked to me anyway. What I didn't realize was that he was also sizing me up, as well, to see if I would accept him as a person and to judge whether I had the potential to learn the craft of Hexerei or Powwow. In the early days, he would make me wait sometimes for an hour at the drugstore in Lexington, South Carolina, until he was ready to visit. I learned later that this was a test of my resolve.

Lee's Hex house was a veritable treasure trove of historical artifacts on this area of South Carolina. An avid bottle collector, he also collected objects that evidenced the spiritual folk-beliefs of the community. In his study, he had many 18th- and 19th-century books that he had found in the Dutch Fork on metaphysical topics from Mesmerism to Druids, as well as Native

American artifacts, local historical memorabilia and pieces of 19th-century furniture decorated with Hex signs as protective measures. He had carved "throw stick" wands, amulets and an old sealed bottle said to contain an incarcerated evil spirit. His combination bedroom and study contained many iron implements, which I learned were employed to diffuse negative psychic energy. Over his bed was a cross, made from the fence that once belonged to a famous witch from the area. In short, he was a man who physically lived immersed in a private world of history and magic.

Lee had a dramatic flair for playful mischief, and behind the door, he had a large black wooden coffin standing upright on a table. He had obtained the coffin from an Odd Fellows Lodge. It contained a small sign bearing the words "Think about it!" just to poke fun at those who might see this reminder of our mortality and be alarmed. In short, the house and atmosphere were steeped in magic. It must be stated that Lee was considered by some in the community to be a Hexenmeister or master witch and denounced by others as a crank and a weirdo. These diverging opinions probably still hold, and Lee would not have minded these labels in the least.

As a genealogist and local historian, Lee had researched Powwow, which he called Hexerei, and concluded that the practice was pre-Christian in origin. He was convinced the tradition was a remnant of the old pagan/Druidic religions of Europe that had originally migrated from the Indian subcontinent. In his local history research, he had traced the movement of German settlers through Pennsylvania, Virginia and into the Carolinas, and he documented the practice of Powwow as it moved with them. In colonial times, the presence of healers and even witches in those early communities were looked upon as a routine part of daily life and a useful resource in times of need. As we know from stories handed down, however, if this resource was seen to have turned upon the community, judgment and punishment were certain and swift.

In most areas where Powwow evolved, it became a sympathetic magic tradition that treats the illness as if personified, and as such can be driven from the body. The words, structure and content of the incantations and traditional hand gestures, such as stroking the person being cured, are vehicles employed to help the practitioner focus his or her mental energy.

Lee taught me that you learn to focus your mind, almost as a photographer focuses a camera. Our thoughts, like our physical selves, are made of energy and are merely in a less-tangible form. Through meditation, prayer and practice, we can learn to give our mental projections additional energy and solidity, allowing them to do the required task. This explains how the Powwow can work successfully with animals and even with plants. "This diversity of potential benefactors of Powwow seems again to challenge the notion that the success of sympathetic healing is based on the faith or the beliefs of the person receiving the treatment, as is sometimes asserted." In his book, *Strange Experience: The Secrets of a Hexenmeister*, Lee tells how "Old Granny Slice, the good witch of Dutch Fork, would start across blazing woodland, and how people marveled when the fire died at her tracks" (120).

These seemingly miraculous events challenge the notion that the success of sympathetic healing is based on the faith or the beliefs of the person receiving the treatment, as is sometimes asserted. In his article entitled "Powwowing among the Pennsylvania Germans," Victor Dieffenbach wrote,

> Some folks do claim that it is a matter of faith or one believes in it. Maybe so; but how about the thousands of poor suffering dumb brutes who have been helped by powwowing? The mule who gets stroked over his body by the hands of some stranger, to relive him of a sore or an attack of colic, does not know that the stroking is to help him in his discomfort. . . . The mule never finds out of having received any treatment whatsoever, yet the result is the same, he gets well, if the person does the right thing. (7)

Lee Gandee's Version of Powwow

Lee Gandee was, in many ways, an atypical Powwow. He was highly educated and an educator himself, whereas most Powwows were farmers or tradesmen. Yet, in other ways, he was a true follower of his magical heritage. Like most Powwows, despite the publishing of his book, Lee was actually secretive about his methods and practice. His magical rituals and incantations had a natural flow. This included how he read the omens and signs of nature, and how he magically employed resources of the natural world, using herbs, trees, water and stones as part of his ritual practice.

Once, when I showed him several items I'd purchased from a mail order occult catalog, he smiled and said, "Do you really think that stuff will help you? Don't you realize by now that the magic is coming from within you and from God? You are the catalyst! In you, the power will either arise or fall flat." He reminded me that, unlike those who claim to confer power via degrees or initiations, "You can either do this [powwow] or you can't. . . . I can only point you in the right direction; you must make it happen. . . . You must make it real . . . and it's no shame if you can't!"

Like most Powwows, Lee Gandee also healed himself. On one occasion, which he mentioned in his book, he treated himself for third-degree burns from an accident with a brush fire. Although he was scared, he said his suffering had been minimal, to the astonishment of his regular physician.

During my time with Lee, the type of healings that fascinated me the most were the ones performed on animals. For example, Lee would receive a phone call from a farmer who was dehorning his cattle and was seeking relief from the bleeding. Lee did not necessarily need to go to the farm to help animals heal. He would call the farmer and conduct the healing by muttering a healing incantation into the telephone. At first, I was astonished by this event, yet when Lee would chant over the telephone, the bleeding would cease.

Powwow and Personal Ethics

Lee knew his legal and personal limits. When he knew his clients also needed conventional medical attention, he advised his clients to see a doctor in addition to seeking his Powwow healing. He never tried to dissuade any of his clients from seeking conventional medical care. Like many Powwows, he viewed his practice as complementary to modern medicine and a manifestation of Divine power in the mundane world. Like other true Powwows, Lee never took money for his services. In older times, however, it was common for a Powwow to find a chicken or bag of flour by his or her door as a token of thanks from a grateful client.

Lee always stressed that managing any sort of knowledge or power, spiritual or otherwise, is a tremendous responsibility. It requires a strongly developed sense of morality, maintaining a personal balance in relation to one's emotions and thoughts and a commitment to ethical behavior. After all, if one's thoughts can actually affect others, the need to control one's thinking becomes critical.

In *Strange Experience*, Lee recounted the story of his great grandfather, who was known for his ability to control the weather. One afternoon, during a storm, his great grandfather became angry at the lightning, which had just struck a favorite tree and frightened his grandson. According to Lee, the old man,

> ...stepped to the edge of the porch, shook his fist at the clouds and cried, "Bust my tree and scare a little boy, damn you! This is old Zach: let's see you flash one at me once!" A Hex should not say such things. The lightening [sic] obeyed him: he was killed instantly. (116).

In the Dutch Fork community where he lived, it was believed that Lee, in a similar moment of anger, had magically injured a young man who had insulted him by wrongfully accusing Lee of stealing peaches. Lee's subsequent curse had destroyed the orchard and caused the mental breakdown of Lee's accuser once he discovered Lee's identity and magical reputation. When questioned about the incident, Lee admitted being angry and cursing the orchard but never admitted to intentionally harming the person. He did express regret that the incident had happened.

The assumption of personal responsibility for one's powers becomes critical when we look at the second major aspect of the practice: that of traveling in, as well as communing with, the spirit world. The level of self-control has to been extended into one's dream life; therefore, learning to control and manipulate one's dreams is one of the first steps in learning Powwow. This technique of dream management and manipulation is now commonly called lucid dreaming.

During my time with Lee, I often heard stories of less than ethical magical practitioners who exploited their clients or otherwise abused their abilities. As Powwows are intermediaries between the spirit world and the world of the embodied, I cannot emphasize enough how strong moral values and ethical behavior are critical to a Powwow's success and personal safety.

Powwows believe that spirits, like their embodied counterparts, have personalities and are found in all phases of personal and spiritual development. One of these ethical values surrounds the types of involvement a magical practitioner will have with spirit beings. For example, there are dangerous taboos about having sexual relations with discarnate entities. Even if initially successful, such a violation of common decency and good commonsense is universally a path to personal disaster and madness.

Humans can increase, consciously or inadvertently, the physical solidity of discarnate spirits through extremes of emotion, such as fear, or by interacting improperly with them. Anyone who plays with this kind of fire will get seriously burned. While some spirits are clearly the psychic residue of human trauma or energy manifestations of formerly embodied humans, others are childlike entities associated with a certain location. The latter are referred to as elementals or nature spirits. One can often sense these nature spirits in woodland settings or near bodies of water. While these nature spirits are usually harmless, others can be very troubled and, like humans, can be treacherous and dangerous to encounter. Such entities should not be approached lightly or alone. Like the old Celtic beliefs in brownies and fairies, these nature spirits can be mischievous and cruel when provoked. We will look at this aspect of Powwow in more detail in the following chapters.

Healing the Physically Sick: The Central Feature of Powwow

Lee followed the traditional Powwow order of healing ailments, which includes:

Interviewing the client: Powwows are known to be excellent listeners and counselors, who are able to pick up the often subtle cues that reveal the physical and emotional components of the complaint. It is believed by Powwows that many physical manifestations of illness actually stem from trauma to the person's mind and spiritual body. Comments like "I just don't feel like myself anymore" or "I feel like the life has been drained out of me" are clear indicators to the Powwow that there could be a trauma-based illness or even magical intrusion from some outside source. Interviewing includes securing the client's full and birth name for use later, as this has value in the treatment phase.

"Reading" the client: This is done in two basic ways: visual and psychic scanning. Sitting across from the client, the Powwow would conduct a visual examination that involved "psychically scanning" the physical body and a person's aura and life energy. This can also be the point at which the Powwow looks for the presence of a magical intrusion. Perhaps the most common method of scanning is to pass the hands over the person's body, without actually touching the client, to get a sense of the field and flow of the client's life energy.

During the scanning process, the physical illness will often present itself as a disruption, an abnormality, and sometimes this experience can be painful to the Powwow. In the 1996 article "Amish 'Voodoo' Applies Belief in Healing Power" by Scott Canon in the *Kansas City Star*, an Amish Braucha, Rachel Smoker of Lancaster County, Pennsylvania, described a healer's sensing such an abnormality this way: "I just feel the pain. . . . I feel the electricity in their bodies" (A10). Often the disruption also comes with a corresponding mental image or intuition to which the Powwow is sensitive and empathetic. "I see the illness in my mind" is how Lee once described this phenomenon of Powwow practice to me.

The point of these first two steps in the tradition of healing is so the Powwow can try to establish a sense of what is normal for that person—to be able to discern any abnormality in that flow. By reading the body's energy field and its movement, the Powwow can also discern, with practice, the cause of the problem and any additional components that may be present. Remember that a traditional healer is addressing the entire person holistically: mentally, emotionally, physically and spiritually. During the examination phase, mental and emotional disturbance would feel to the Powwow like a hole or emptiness near the person's heart. A magical intrusion feels alien or as though it does not belong inside the body or consciousness.

Lee understood that people became injured spiritually through traumatic events like a death, incest, rape, assault, physical injury or other major life disruptions. Even the act of childbirth, if traumatic, can produce this sort of loss of or injury to one's life energy.

Modern psychology has many terms for this sort of illness, including depression, post-traumatic stress disorder and post-partum depression. I once heard of a veteran of the Vietnam War who went to a Powwow for his psychic wounds after returning home, because he could not deal with the memories of his wartime experiences. This Powwow treated this man successfully over a period of six months to restore his sense of emotional well-being by retrieving those mental constructs that had become separated from his personality because of the war.

Lee frequently said that we were, at our essence, one with God, but that our personality in this life was a collection of mental constructs that have evolved because we have taken on a physical form to directly interact with the outer world. These constructs form an inherently fragile coalition that serves us with varying degrees of success. It is those constructs that we are healing—not our essence—which is unchanging and merely a witness to our existence.

Anthropologists have identified this particular shamanic therapy as "soul retrieval." At the request of the client, the shaman goes into a trance, enters the spirit realm, locates and retrieves the fragmented mental constructs and returns them to the client. The shaman then reassembles and restores this person's life energy or soul, which has become, in shamanic terms, fragmented or lost by the trauma.

Performing the healing: This is generally accomplished through a ritual that may include: softly chanting a charm, while touching the client with the hands or with a twig or stone to draw out the inflammation or fever; or use of the breath in a blowing or sucking manner to cool a wound or withdraw an illness, followed by a quick exhalation. This temporary "taking in" of an illness is somewhat unique to Powwow, and is described by Ralph R. Kuna, in the *Mankind Quarterly* article, "Hoodoo: The Indigenous Medicine and Psychiatry of the Black American":

> The powwower will frequently draw the disorder from the patient's body into his own. The powwower in effect "takes on" (absorbs) the illness of the patient. This is something no Hoodoo doctor would consider doing. (142)

As an additional ritual of detection, some Powwows may take a measure of the person with a piece of string. This practice can be used to get a sense of the person's energy, and in some procedures, the string can be used to draw the negative element from the client's body. This ritual extraction and absorption of an illness may also include the patient being walked through or passed through a natural hole in a tree or stone to "pull" the illness away from the client into a foreign object. I once witnessed a fever being ritually transferred to an ordinary hen's egg, which later, upon being cracked open, appeared as black bile instead of its normal color.

As for incantations, they are almost always repeated three times or in multiples of three. A recent email informant called "Stovepipe" relayed the old German saying with regard to placing a hex or curse on a person: "3 to make 'em ill, 6 to lay 'em down and 9 to knock 'em." The use of the number three, according to Raven Grimassi in the *Encyclopedia of Wicca and Witchcraft,* is based on a magical principle called the Triangle of Manifestation, which says,

> This basic principle is rooted in the number of three. It is a metaphysical belief that in order to manifest something, three components must come together. These components are time, space, and energy. The functioning of the components is such that if a time and a space are selected into which energy is directed, a manifestation will occur. (375-376)

It must be restated that the process of ritual in Powwow is designed to facilitate and conduct a movement of Divine energy through the vehicle of the Powwow into or out of the client. The adult human clients of the healing have, even at the unconscious level, some expectation of the effectiveness of the healing. This expectation provides an added receptivity to the movement of Divine energy. Hence, the healing will, if conducted properly, result in an internal response and manifest as a restoration of the client's multilevel system of health. The Powwow and client are, in essence, actors in the process. "God is all there is," Lee often said, "Satan was a lie from the beginning!"

A Powwow will also go into a trance that, along with the words and gestures, may appear outwardly pointless, yet they are understood to facilitate the internal manifestation or movement of this energy. The movement of the internal energy is what actually facilitates the healing.

With regard to their content and structure, incantations appear to follow no established pattern, except for the benediction at the end. Here's an example from John George Hohman's *The Long Lost Friend* that I learned for the treatment of bruises. Hands positioned over the bruised area, one should say three times:

Bruise thou shalt not heat,
Bruise thou shalt not sweat,
Bruise thou shalt not run,
No more than the Virgin Mary shall bring forth another son.
God the father, God the Son, and God the Holy Ghost.

Often an incantation is repeated several times using the person's name as part of the incantation. In the famous Powwow chapbook entitled, *Secrets of Sympathy,* by William Wilson Beissel, the author says, "If the patient is very sick or has severe pain the sympathy may be repeated every 15 or 30 minutes for three times or offener [sic] as the condition and case demand" (32). Here is one of Beissel's sympathies for fever:

> For Fever mention the sick person's Christian name three times, and then say the following words each time:

> Heaven and earth were created, and all was good, all that is made of God is good; only the fever is a vexation; therefore avert from me, leave me, go away, disappear before me. Thou shalt flee upon high mountains, thou shalt move into the abyss, go out from me in the name of John, the Holy Apostle, and Jesus Christ, the son of God. (41)

Many Powwows also finish by making the sign of the cross with the right hand curled into a fist, thumb pointing downward. Lee indicated this hand position was a symbolic two-fold gesture of blessing the client and attacking the illness. A Holy stone (also called a Holey stone), a stone with a natural hole or a stone specially prepared for healing may also be employed to draw the illness from the client's body in an act of magical transference.

During my research with Lee, I have not personally seen him heal with a Holey Stone but have observed other Powwows employing it to remove pain and inflammation. The hole becomes a channel through which the pain is psychically withdrawn. Like many of the tools employed in Powwow, the object is simply a vehicle to aid and focus the healer's energy.

Concluding the healing: To conclude the healing, Powwows will symbolically sweep the illness and any other negative energy from the client's body. To do this, the Powwow will perform a systematic brushing motion over the person's body, toward the floor. Prayers that the client can hear

and understand usually follow the brushing. The 23rd Psalm and the Lord's
Prayer were routinely used for this purpose.

It is interesting to note that with the presence of the neopagan and
Goddess spiritual traditions, other holy names are being employed in the
place of the Christian ones by non-Christian Powwows. I've heard the one
mentioned above for bruises completed with the phrase "In the name of
the Maiden, the Mother and the Crone," with the same rate of success.
Fortunately, for all of us, the Divine is beyond our feeble attempts to name
or lay claim to its favor. The Divine can also hear our prayers no matter
what name or form we assign to it. It is abundantly clear to me that no
one religious group or nation has the exclusive franchise to the Divine's
mercy and grace.

Curing the "Verhexed" or Removal of Magical Intrusions

During my association with Lee, I observed how frequently neighbors and
others who had learned of his abilities to conduct healings and other services called upon him. They usually came in secret, asking that no one in
the community be informed of their visit. One of the ritual services they
commonly requested of Lee was called a "take off" or removal of a magical intrusion. Signs of an intrusion of this sort would include the person
suddenly feeling strangely ill or mentally oppressed, experiencing strange
nightmares, a sense of personal disorientation and emotional disassociation
with normal everyday life. Any or all of these can be signs of someone's
negative magic or the intrusion of something in the living or spirit world
into their lives.

In his book, *Strange Experience*, Lee records a request for help from a
Dutch Fork neighbor, noting that he "was startled when she flatly stated that
someone had placed a witch-crab in her stomach to devour her vitals and
kill her" (322). This particular form of magical intrusion, which had taken
the form of a mental construct, is actually more common to Hoodoo than
to Powwow, so Lee's therapy adopted and adapted the Hoodoo practice of
using graveyard dirt or "goofer-dust" over a nine-day period to drive the
magical entity out of her body. Lee said the client claimed to have "glimpsed
it as it passed out onto the ground and scurried off" (323).

As will be shown in the interviews with Lee Gandee, the afflicted person, family members or friends would call Lee to explain the nature of the problem and arrange an appointment with him. One interesting aspect of removing a bad spell that is common to all three traditions, Hex, Hoodoo and Powwow, was the need to identify the source of the negative spell or hex. Paul Frazier, in his article, "Some Lore of Hexing and Powwowing," in *Midwest Folklore,* echoes this initial step when he says a "braucher begins his cure by finding the hexer" (103).

As in the practice of Hoodoo, knowing the source of the magical intrusion allows the Powwow to ritually remove or "take off" the intrusion and send it back to the person or thing from which it originated. Ritually, this involved circling the victim, who was seated in a chair, and chanting a certain incantation three times in sequence. As noted before, this employment of repetitions of three and the use of holy names is an essential element in a Powwow's ability to remove a hex, spell and/or magical intrusion.

Here is such an incantation from another Powwow spell book, *Albertus Magnus or Egyptian Secrets,* named after a Dominican friar, known as Saint Albert the Great, who wrote extensively on topics such as astrology and magic in the 13th century. This was employed to remove the effects of an evil spirit:

> Thou arch-sorcerer, thou has attacked (complete name); let that witchcraft recede from him into thy marrow and into thy bone, let it be returned unto thee. I exorcise thee for the sake of the five wounds of Jesus, thou evil spirit, and conjure thee for the five wounds of Jesus of this flesh, marrow and bone; I exorcise thee for the sake of the five wounds of Jesus, at this very hour restore to health again N. N., in the name of God the Father, God the Son, and of God the Holy Spirit. Three times. (5)

Here is another incantation, directly translated by Joseph H. Peterson from the original, famous German medieval text, *Romanus-Büchlein: vor Gott der Herr bewahre meine Seele, meinen Aus- und Eingang; von nun an bis in alle Ewigkeit, Amen. Halleluja. (Little Book of the Roma, Before God the Lord Preserve My Soul, My Going and Coming; from Now to All Eternity, Amen. Halleluja.)*

> To prevent being Cheated, Charmed, or Bewitched and to be at all times blessed. [H 161]
> Like unto the cup, and the wine, and the holy supper, which our dear

Lord Jesus Christ gave unto his dear disciples on Maundy Thursday, may
the Lord Jesus guard me in day time, and at night, that no dog may bite
me, no wild beast tear me to pieces, no tree fall on me, no water rise
against me, no fire-arms injure me, no weapons, no steel, no iron cut me,
no fire burn me, no false sentence fall upon me, no false tongue injure
me, no rogue enrage me, and that no fiends, no witchcraft and enchantment can harm me. Amen.

To Release Spell-bound Persons. [H 136]
You horseman and footman, whom I here conjured at this time, you may
pass on in the name of Jesus Christ, through the word of God and the
will of Christ; ride ye on now and pass.

Often the client's face and hands would also be washed in water or his
body magically swept to remove the negative psychic energy. At the end of
the ritual, the victim would be given a protective charm and/or instructed
on what to do should the intrusion recur. This protective action is a magical process known as warding. Lee, as we shall see later, was very gifted at
this practice.

The final aspect of removing magical intrusions was the practice of
magically "binding" the person causing the problem. Binding involved a
counter-spell created, energized and sent back along the energy trail left by
the original intrusion. This part of the process, without doing any physical
or mental injury to the individual, effectively enclosed or bound them from
sending further malice toward the client or anyone else. To bind, Lee, having
identified the source, would mentally project the binding while chanting
the binding spell. Often the person targeted by this binding would become
psychically incapacitated and would eventually call or visit Lee to apologize
for the mischief and promise not to do so again.

I experienced a similar situation myself as my magical reputation became
public after I gave several talks on Powwow and Hexerei. After a poorly
written newspaper account of my thesis research while I was a student at the
University of South Carolina, there was an incident with an overly ambitious
Huna (traditional Hawaiian shaman), who visited me in a college classroom
and proceeded to psychically attack me. The Huna later apologized to my
professor. See Chapter 8 for details of this encounter.

Binding as a form of response certainly seems more humane than some responses employed against malevolent spell-casters in the past. Such a ritual was used recently by a family of Powwows living near Philadelphia to respond to the sexual assault of one of their younger female relatives. While the rapist was never formally charged and certainly never apologized, he has not been able to effectively escape the results of his actions. He is now lodged in the state prison for an identical crime, where he will come to personally understand the type of pain that his crime inflicted on a child. In this case, the entire family gathered and focused their energy on rendering him incapable of escaping the effects of his actions. Such binding involves mentally encapsulating the offending individual through visualization of the event and ritually binding an object representing the offender with a string or ribbon or similar item. This sympathetic magic is a way of tricking the ordinary mind into projecting its energy toward a specified target. The object itself is only a point of focus and may be a doll or even a potato, which was used in this particular ritual. The potato, in this case, was buried under a tree near the cemetery, as a way of sealing the spell. In this particular spell-casting, family spirits were summoned from the cemetery to aid the process of transmission and contribute their energy to the process. Other Powwows not living in the area were called and told when and how to join in the process.

Another way for a Powwow to cast a spell of binding or other magical action involves the practice of creating a paper charm, whereupon the name of the person to be bound is written. The paper is rolled and tied with red cord. The charm should then be psychically charged and sealed within a hole you have bored in a tree known for protection and strength, such as an oak or willow. After inserting the rolled charm into the hole, a plug from the tree or one you have created is used to seal the hole and complete the spell. One will notice that this is similar in intent to a ritual where a witch bottle or jar is used to contain and set the spell. I have seen trees in the Dutch Fork of South Carolina, in Virginia and in Pennsylvania that have been employed in such a manner. To release the binding or spell, the plug is removed and the charm destroyed. See the Appendix for more details about the creation and use of charms.

The Complementary Relationship between Incantations, Herbs, Objects and Rituals in the Making of Magical Charms

Another aspect of the practice of Powwow is the knowledge and use of herbs in the various healings and protective measures performed by the Hex. Powwows have often been master herbalists, who learned over a lifetime how to use what grew naturally around them for medicinal purposes. As for incantations and rituals, there were even guidebooks like Hohman's *The Long Lost Friend,* or *The Sixth and Seventh Books of Moses* (author and source unknown) and *Albertus Magnus.* Friar Albertus Magnus provided recipes for potions and plasters, along with spells for all manner of purposes from colic in horses to spellbinding thieves to curing snakebite to banishment of evil spirits. Many of these books were compilations of charms and spells from many sources.

In *American Folk Medicine: A Symposium,* Don Yoder's chapter, "Hohman and Romanus: Origins and Diffusion of the Pennsylvania German Powwow Manual," traces many of the charms and incantations found in *The Long Lost Friend* to the aforementioned 18th-century German spell book, the *Romanus-Büchlein.* Yoder says that *The Long Lost Friend* "became the leading charm collection for the German-speaking countries of Europe, where it is still in print and in use" (238). While Lee Gandee had an extensive knowledge of herbs and their properties, I rarely saw Lee employ herbs in his practice. One exception was in the making of protective charms, such as a cross made of vervain, which was hung in a window or over a door to repel magical intrusions. I believe he knew that giving clients herbal potions was like walking a legal tightrope.

Finding Missing or Stolen Items

A second type of Lee's practice involved the discovery and identification of someone who had stolen a possession belonging to the client. Lee relates one such encounter in his book, *Strange Experience,* where a potential thief was caught in a magical trap at the doorstep of a house he intended to burgle. He remained magically frozen, unable to move or respond, until released by the owners of that home.

Paul Frazier, in "Some Lore of Hexing and Powwowing," relates a similar incident, where a braucher thwarted a robbery by temporarily paralyzing the thief:

> A robber once stole a team and wagon. But he was captured by a braucher who simply walked three times around the team and wagon. The robber was unable to free himself; finally, according to my informant, the braucher released him by walking three times. (104)

Magical Private Investigation

This portion of Lee's practice involved searching for information on the activities or whereabouts of a person with whom the client had lost contact or suspected of some misdeed—usually infidelity. After interviewing the client, Lee would employ trance and go in search of the missing individual. Another method Lee used was scrying, or visual divination, by looking into a mirror or bowl of water. In true shamanic fashion, the Hex will project his own consciousness, first into the realm of spirits, and then to the place in question. Often Lee would call forth and send a familiar spirit entity known and trusted by him to secure the needed information. He would often send his spirits on such missions because sending his own consciousness at his age was exhausting.

Only experience and a strong commitment to ethical behavior will protect the Powwow during this hazardous effort. He or she will be vulnerable, by this heightened state of awareness, to magical intrusions by a living person or predatory incursions and possible possession by a spirit entity. For example, Lee would enter trance by lying on his bed. To protect himself, he would wear certain amulets, such as a Holey stone. On occasion, Lee would ask me or someone else he trusted to watch over him, with instructions for specific protective actions to be taken, should certain signs appear and trouble arise. Signals that trouble was afoot would include painful moaning, convulsive shaking similar to an epileptic seizure, hyperventilation, eyes wide open but not comprehending what is seen and vocalizing in a strange, unfamiliar voice. The person guarding the Powwow in trance must be ready to spring into action with prayers, blessed water and iron implements to lay upon the body, with a fearless attitude toward the intruder.

Hex Signs: Symbolic Prayers

Along with the magical charm, another magical device Lee regularly created and employed was the Hex sign. His creations were beautiful and highly personalized. The concept of making magical designs and surrounding them with a circle goes far back in human history.

Lee described the Hex sign as a form of painted prayer and wrote in *Strange Experience*,

> The uniformly gratifying outcome of these hex prayers has left me with the feeling that while verbal prayer is adequate for many things, painted prayers are far more certain to accomplish their purpose. (312)

Lee continued,

> All my personal experience suggests that magical power is derived from the action of the mind at the deeper, subconscious level, beneath the cognitive mind to the source of life itself. A symbol is more potent that a naturalistic representation simply because a realistic drawing is interpreted mainly at the conscious level. (312)

These colorful, stylized Hex symbols have reached such popularity with the mainstream culture that they can be purchased in craft shows and are often created by people who may have no idea of their original intended use.

In the article entitled, "The Story of the Hex Sign," which appeared in the *Amish Country News*, Brad Igou says, "The earliest documented hex signs on barns date back to the later half of the 19th century, perhaps because barns weren't generally painted at all much before 1830" (par. 4).

Hex signs as barn decorations did not appear in the Pennsylvania Dutch areas of Pennsylvania in any real numbers until after 1950, according to David Fooks, in "The History of Hex Signs," published in the *Pennsylvania German Review*. Hex signs were popularized by Johnny Ott and Jacob Zook, two Pennsylvania Dutch artists, whose works can still be purchased in tourist and online stores. Before the 1950s, Hex signs as magical creations were placed on items within the home such as furniture and books. In the Dutch Fork of South Carolina, examples of this sort of furniture decoration can still be seen in private homes and at the Lexington County Museum. These Hex items were meant to be private expressions of personal needs, not for public display, until very recent times.

Social Invisibility and Eccentricity as Personal Protection

In South Carolina during the early 1970s, Powwow was unknown to the general community that had grown around the Dutch Folk during the late 1950s and 1960s. Outside of certain families, Powwow was not spoken of in public or in polite company, or was publicly denounced as being the province of the superstitious or the mentally unstable. Families who practiced Powwow also performed the art of social invisibility, blending seamlessly into their communities. For practicing families, this type of magical tradition was considered a gift from God and not to be exhibited as a public demonstration. According to Lee and others I met during my field research, many of the old-timers in the Dutch Fork were angry with Lee for being so audacious and disrespectful as to write a book about his magical practice. They were concerned that it would make them appear superstitious and reflect negatively on the community.

The average person won't find Powwows unless they choose to reveal themselves. Lee, on the other hand, claimed he was not ashamed of the term Powwow, or even witch, although he would have surely found some of the modern neopagan expressions of magical practice amusing—with their initiations, strict hierarchy and coven rules. To Lee, the craft of the wise was a way of life, as natural as breathing and simply a way of responding to the world around him.

During my years of study with him, Lee swore me to many secrets concerning the practice of Powwow. "You don't need to go tell everyone you know, what you know," he said. "They don't have the ears to hear you! Give it [Powwow] some time to settle in before you go talking about it! Most of this old world is still going to think you are out of your mind. That is your protection."

Lee would often make absurd statements or ramble on, until those watching him were convinced of his insanity and harmlessness. Once I became really angry with him over this. After he gave a public lecture, he began to ramble during the question and answer session.

"Why did you do that?" I demanded. "Now those folks will think you're just some crazy old man!"

"I want them to," Lee quietly replied. "Did you see those two men in the back of the room? I realized that they were there to determine whether or not I was for real and were intending to approach me about working spells for them. They were dangerous characters, so I let them think I'm crazy. Better that than having to deal with them. If they thought you and I were for real, we would not be safe."

"I understand," I replied.

"Good." He smiled as he lit his pipe. "Remember, a crazy man has nothing to explain and no one wants anything to do with him." It became clear to me at that moment that Powwow is not a path for those needing fame or recognition.

Lee's Pupil Goes "Native"

The healing aspect of Powwow was one that I realized I could easily learn and adapt to my own life. I soon started healing burns, stopping blood, and taking away pain for myself and for others. The appearance of, and working with, the spirit world, and in particular the visible manifestations of non-physical entities, was personally very unsettling for me in the early days. It has taken years to develop a comfortable relationship with the presence of this alternate reality.

Lee protected me at first and would tell me that I had "just imagined it" or "just pay it no mind, it's not going to hurt you." For me, this was what he was referring to when he talked about "being able to manage it."

I found it very difficult to move between the world of everyday life and the states of being Lee revealed and helped me to achieve. It was like having to return to your quiet little hometown after you've been living or traveling in some exotic land. Everything may look the same, but you have changed, and nothing feels as it did before you began your journey.

To my distress, Lee once said, "I'm afraid I can't help you. If you're going to walk this road, it will exact a price from you. You can no more go back to your ordinary world than you can go back to being a child again, no matter how you may try. . . . You can only accept what has happened and keep growing."

As with all true spiritual paths, magical or otherwise, there comes a point, an epiphany and a moment in which your perceptions change forever and the transformation begins.

Lee was not a man possessed of extraordinary personal arrogance or an inflated sense of his magical power. "I'm just like everyone else," he said one afternoon. "I sometimes behave badly. I'm given to my desires and betrayed by my needs." He loved his family, was proud of his children—even in their struggles—and expressed great regret about the pain he caused them by the public revelation, in his book, of his homosexuality. He was especially sad at the pain he'd caused his former wife. "She is a good woman," he remarked one day. "I wish I could have spared her all of this."

To me, Lee demonstrated that even those who have found and follow a spiritual path still must often walk upon rocky ground. Finding a spiritual path is a light in the woods, but you're still going to occasionally wander through the thickets.

Sadly, Lee passed from this plane of existence on October 10, 1998, in West Columbia, South Carolina, at the age of 81. We had not spoken for many years, as our paths were only meant to cross for that short time of four years. Sometimes, however, when I listen to the old tapes I made of our talks (the ones he allowed the recorder to record!), I believe I can feel his presence. Why shouldn't I? Memory is a powerful presence and the world of spirit occupies the same space and time as our own.

Lee often noted that spirits are all around us, all the time. It is simply a matter of altering your perception and they are there. He once said, "At your center is God . . . what you've been seeking all through your many lifetimes. You are not apart from it (the Divine) . . . and you can never be. It is you. What you see in this life is like a dream! It's a combination of your imperfect senses interacting with your limited mind . . . but the ultimate reality is right there." Then he would point to me, and add, "You just have to awaken to its presence and nothing will ever be the same again . . . I promise you!"

He was right, although I didn't fully understand the depth of his statements at the time. The path of the Powwow or any other shamanic practice can be arduous, if not dangerous, at times; but it is a compelling mystery, a journey of self-discovery, of learning just who and what you really are. The best part is that it never ends! That revelation to me is such a comfort and joy in this ongoing, wonderful process. There is no end to our soul's journey, as we are always in a process of becoming, whether in this corporeal state or beyond. There's also no need to be afraid of physical death, as there is too much wonder ahead of you. I'm sure that somewhere, somehow, Lee is still on his path, still wandering the expanse of endless time and space. I just may catch up with him one day. The following chapters include a few of my interviews and adventures with this marvelous individual.

CHAPTER FIVE

My First Interview with the Hexenmeister

The beginning of knowledge is the discovery of something we do not understand.
—Frank Herbert (1920–1986)

We make our own reality out of what we believe.   —Lee Gandee, 1974

"HOW DOES ONE BECOME a Hexenmeister?" I asked him at our first meeting.

"By being a Hex until he can manage it!"

The tall, distinguished gentleman had greeted me cordially and led me to a large study decorated with a number of pictures, an extensive bottle collection and a large wooden cross over the rope bed where I learned he slept. There was a coffin propped up against a short bookcase in the corner behind the door. We settled into rocking chairs, and he lit his ever-present pipe.

JM: I'm really interested in your personal history and how you came to be involved in all of this.

LG: How did you find me?

JM: I spent a summer in the library trying to research as much as I could about the topic, and then I found someone who had heard of you. I then went to the library and read your article in *Sandlapper* and decided that it was extremely relevant to the paper and what I was studying.

He then asked me what other research I had done. I spoke of the time I spent with Mr. McTeer and the root-doctor culture around Beaufort.

LG: I believe Dr. Buzzard is dead, isn't he? All of the old root doctors are dead except for Mr. McTeer. Ms. Cannon is doing a study of root doctors in Georgia. She is quite knowledgeable. You should try to find her.

JM: People often come to the likes of Mr. McTeer for psychic help and counseling. Do they come to you as well?

LG: They come to me and I try to put them off as best I can, 'cause they're always trying to get me to put something on somebody's husband or somebody's wife or something like that, and I'm just not interested in that. By the way, have you read my book?

JM: No, but I plan to. Where do you think all of this practice came from?

LG: I may have made a mistake in thinking this area was settled by Germans. The area was mostly Swiss, but they were still German in the sense that they were Germanic people. You see, the Saxe-Gotha Township was set up in 1736 as a buffer against a possible French invasion from the Alabama territory at Mobile and between themselves and the Native American Indian tribes of the upcountry, including the Cherokee. King George II wanted to attract Germans because they were most reliable and could be counted upon to hold the land, if they were attacked, until help could come from Charleston.

As he named the pattern of counties laid out in colonial South Carolina, he reminded me that those settlements were to be a buffer against the English settlements on the coast, which at that time were centered around Charleston and Beaufort.

LG: George II paid out of his private funds to have a booklet published in Gall, Switzerland, in 1740, and a man who had lived in Saxe-Gotha Township went back to Switzerland and scattered these booklets all up and down the Rhine River in both Switzerland and Germany, although the English colonial government particularly wanted the Swiss. The immigrants who came founded the Saxe-Gotha settlement, which was located on the river below Cayce [West Columbia, South Carolina]. It never did turn into a town, but there was a fort there.

The first fort in Lexington [South Carolina], and a trading post, was built in 1718. It had a garrison of twenty men. Two Native American tribes, the Cherokees and the Congrees, would come to the post to trade. To the Indians it was neutral territory where two main foot routes—one running north and south, the other east and west—met at the river.

JM: How and where did the art of the Hexenmeister develop?

I was trying to move the conversation away from a review of social and political history.

LG: That is still—unless it has been done in Europe and I don't know about it—still to be figured out, but there are some indications based on a recently published book called *The Bog People*. It includes a picture of the ceremonial silver Gundestrup Cauldron [found in a Danish peatbog in 1891] that was associated with the religious ceremonies conducted there, which were Druid, I suppose. The workmanship of this vessel was considered to be eastern Celtic and one of the designs on that cauldron shows the hex sign, which is on the cover of my book already, as a sacred symbol. On that same cauldron were two elephants, suggesting that the symbol came out of Africa or Asia. I believe it came from India originally, and I think there has been a big mistake in the definition of the word "hex." You see, in Hexerei, the number six is extremely important. You know, with the six days of creation and so on, and there are supposed to be six steps to follow in any work you do in Hexerei. Those six petals of the rosette are symbolic in a number of invocations. The Greek word for six is "hex" and I think the word "hex" refers to the number six rather than to the German word Hexe, or witch. People who do not "practice powwow" realized that people who "employ"—"use" this particular healing art—can do things that you normally think of as witchcraft. They then developed the German word *Hexe* from this association.

JM: So, you think it came from India?

LG: I think it came from the same system that produced the Indian religions. It's very similar to some of the Indian religions. It believes in reincarnation, believes in an over soul, that all life is interconnected and conscious to a degree. If you are conscious, so are the trees, so are the rocks, etc.

JM: I am also studying Asian religions, and I have noticed the use of sacred symbols in Asian art.

LG: Mandalas. Of course, the Gundestrup sign serves the same purpose as the Mandala. Both concentrate the attention and perform a certain function on the subconscious mind, because it has to do certain internal things so the mind can follow the pattern. It has to balance itself, for example. You're looking at a cross, a Greek cross, which is a Hex cross in that it is square. Anything geometric does something to balance the conscious mind, that's its purpose. It draws the conscious mind into a state of balance. If you look at a perfectly balanced geometric design, with half above and half below, it draws things into a balance. That's what we want to be, we want to be balanced people. The Hex believes that body and soul are just part of the same thing: The outer picture of the soul forms the body, and the body needs to be in good condition for the soul to be in good condition. That's rather sound thinking, I'd say.

JM: You indicated earlier in the article about you in the *Sandlapper* magazine that you are not a South Carolina native but came from West Virginia. You also said that the practice was in your family. Could you elaborate on this?

LG: You'll find a great deal of information about my background in my book, in the chapter called "The Daugherty Influence."

Lee then relayed a story about being born under a cloud of suspicion [as to his paternity], which resulted in his being raised by a surrogate grandmother who had, he believed, "engineered the whole thing" so that, in the ensuing confusion, she would be able to take the baby.

LG: She took me when I was six months old, and she wasn't really my grandmother because she had adopted my mother. So, I grew up with this other family, who were Daughertys, an Irish name. That family goes back to the 1760s in western Virginia. They were massacred by

Indians at a place called Meadowcreek, which is in Greenbriar, West Virginia, except for one boy who was taken in and raised by a German family as a German. And his grandson eventually returned to western Virginia. He was known to draw Pennsylvania designs and magical designs and the like, although he always used English as his language rather than German. His family prided themselves in having some knowledge of Hexerei. They could contact spirits, see apparitions, had knowledge of what was going to happen or knowledge of what was going on in another location. My "grandmother" was the one who had perhaps the strongest faith, saying she could command things to happen. I got to the point as a child that, if I wanted something to happen, I would try to do as she did. And it would happen.

She [Lee's "grandmother"] practiced stopping blood when people got cut. When I was just a little kid on the floor, I can remember people calling her on the phone saying that their child had stepped on broken glass and was bleeding real bad and would she please "use" to stop it. She would mutter something over the phone and say to call back if it didn't stop immediately. It worked on animals as well as people. If a farmer was dehorning cattle and the cattle bled, he would call. Then she would ask, "What color is it? When was it born?" and so on. She would tell the farmer to say a particular verse from the Bible and the bleeding would stop.

When I asked my late maternal grandmother whether she had ever heard of such things, this utterly pragmatic, practical, deeply religious individual replied, "Of course. My father, your great-grandfather, was such a man. He was especially good at curing animals. People from miles around would send for him to see to their cow or horse or dog." My grandmother viewed such things as a gift of God and called the ability to perform such feats "a blessing" and a confirmation of properly applied Christian faith.

Lee's Background and Magical Upbringing

LG: Watching my grandmother gave me the childhood feeling that all you need to know is the right words to say and you can do things. Then

I started finding out that other people could cure burns, stop certain diseases through a ritual event involving a thread or a piece of paper with your name written on it. Then I learned that the Pennsylvania Dutch in Pennsylvania have Braucherei, Hexerei, and all sorts of things that they use.

JM: There's a woman in Sumter (South Carolina) who has been documented to be able to "speak" a burn off your hand.

LG: Well, I had a terrible burn several years ago . . . that happened here.

He indicated his current home and then showed me some rather horrific scars from third-degree burns on the underside of his arms. He had been burning trash when the fire went out of control. When he realized he was badly burned, he said to his daughter that he wished he knew someone who could "use" for the burns. She suggested he try it on himself, and so he went inside, faced a mirror and said the spell.

LG: Something happened. I took a chill that felt like I'd been touched with dry ice and from that time on until right now, the burns haven't hurt a bit. I put sulfur and dried powdered alum on it as the skin began to fall off in pieces the size of a half-dollar. I put my shirt back on and kept the burns clean.

Several months later, the family doctor, upon seeing the scars, was aghast at their severity and asked Lee how he had been able to withstand the pain. When Lee remarked that he had "used sympathy," the doctor was amazed.

JM: Is "using" still practiced in this area?

LG: Oh, yes, take a person my age and older, and one person in five "uses" for something. There's a fellow about your age, lives over near here and goes to the University of South Carolina who "uses." Mike's his name. I taught him a little bit about Hexerei. When he recently went to his friend's house, he found a dog that had been run over and was unable to get up. His friend was sure the dog was going to die. Mike "used" for him and by the time he left the dog had gotten up and was eating. The next time he saw it, the dog was out playing. So, it worked for broken bones on that dog.

JM: Do you think the folks around here have been doing it for a long time?

LG: I know for a fact they've been doing it for over a hundred and fifty years, because the women who taught me about the burns was about eighty, and she'd learned it from her mother and so on. So, over in Dutch Fork, they've "used" ever since the settlement.

JM: Amazing!

LG: It's not amazing at all! There's supposed to be sixty thousand or more recognized witches in Germany at the present time [1974] and almost all of them are "users." So, it's perfectly logical that they'd "use" in the old days. They had no medicine and they knew it worked. And what you want is something that works when you need it.

Here's one of the old sayings (a cure for the "schlear" a swelling of the glands in the jaw):

Der Schlear und der Drach, Gingen mit einander über'm Bach:
Der Schlear sich verdrank; Und der Drach verswand.
Gott, der Vater, Gott, der Sohn; Und Gott, der heilige Geist; Amen.

And here's what it means in English:

The schlear and the dragon
Went together over the brook:
The schlear was drowned;
And the dragon disappeared.
God, the Father; God, the Son; And God the Holy Ghost. Amen.

I have also found an exact copy of this chant in *A Carolina Dutch Fork Calendar: Manner and Customs in the Olden Times,* by James Everett Kibler, Jr., published by the Dutch Fork Press in 1988.

That's been said in Dutch Fork since the settlement, and to translate doesn't make a lick of sense.

He then read to me an excerpt from an article by author John Hawkins who stated in his 1907 article for *Popular Science Monthly,* "Magical Medical Practice in South Carolina" that people of the

German settlement of South Carolina still held to their traditional beliefs in healing, and he traced these beliefs to their pre-Christian origins. As Hawkins indicates,

> In old Germany neither Charlemagne's conquest nor the priest that followed it could put a period to the use of staves carved with mystic runes and devoted to the purposes of divination and incantation. The oak, the ash, and the willow preserved their sacred character; and in the old heathen formulas used for the cure of disease, the only change effected by Christianity was the substitution of the 'three highest names' (Father, Son, and Holy Ghost) for those of Thor, Woden and other heathen deities. (171)

Hawkins illustrates this cultural incorporation by giving the pagan and then Christian form of a well-known incantation for the healing of sprains:

Pagan version:

> Phol and Woden went to the wood, there was Balder's colt his foot wrenched,
> Then Sinthgunt charmed it and Sunna her sister,
> Then Frua charmed it and Volla her sister, the woden charmed it as he well could, as well the bone-wrench,
> as the joint wrench,
> as the blood-wrench,
> bone to bone,
> blood to blood,
> joint to joint,
> as if they were glued together.

Christian version:

> Our Lord rode, his foal's foot slade,
> Down he lighted, his foal's foot righted,
> Bone to bone,
> Sinew to sinew,
> Flesh to flesh,
> Heal, in the name of the Father, the Son, and the Holy Ghost.
> Amen. (Hawkins 171)

JM: How do you account for the fact that it works? Is it like the Hindu mantra? Is it the power of the words themselves?

LG: Well, for some, words are the power of suggestion. In Hex, whatever a person believes is true, for him. We make our own reality out of what we believe. So, that's the secret of witchcraft in a very few words. That's the secret of witchcraft, and the more you believe that, the stronger a witch you are.

JM: I know that one of my basic conclusions from what is going on in Beaufort is that Mr. McTeer and a few others are practicing a form of or a combination of counseling and rituals that sometimes seem made up, appearing downright hokey, but it works! Most of the clients seem to be suffering from marital or other personal problems and come to the root doctors for treatment they trust, administered by someone they trust. Often it all seems like a grand show of some sort. I once saw McTeer draw a spirit out of a person and it seemed like some sort of a magic trick involving flash powder triggered by his foot. I was watching closely.

LG: *[smiling]* Oh, yes. A lot of times it has to be that way. I performed a magic ceremony for a couple who were undergoing some terrible physical persecution at the time. One of them was about to die from it. My ceremony worked just beautifully, although I made up my own ritual as I went, and I used the names of trees in Latin as part of my incantation. I also took a boy along for power as he was scared to death, and I could use that terror as my emotional stimulus. You have to have some emotional stimulus to make this stuff come to life and work. But the outcome almost paralyzed me.

See, we need salt in the ceremony, and the people were afraid that an evil spirit would come into the house that night and bother them. So, I made a circle of salt around the front steps and told them that anything with bad intentions couldn't cross the salt. They went to bed that night scared to death and waited for something to happen. Well, about one o'clock in the morning one of their neighbors, who lived across the creek, for some reason came over, and when he got to the bottom step where the salt was, he had his foot ready to step up and found he couldn't move it. He couldn't set it down and he was just standing there, one foot raised in the air. So, the dogs rushed out ready to jump on him.

The woman woke up and woke her husband, who opened the door to find the neighbor standing there in a trance of some sort. The woman then remembered that if you touch someone and say, "In the name of John the Baptist, I command you to come out of this state," it breaks the spell. So, they gathered around the man, touched him and said, "In the name of John the Baptist, wake up!" The man came to, but did not know who or where he was even though he was their neighbor. He ended up paying them a dollar to tell him who he was and to take him home. My friend said they took the man to his sister's house and you could hear him carrying on like a crazed man the rest of the night.

According to the old belief, if they had not touched him and the sun had come up, it would have killed him right there where he stood. So, that's what it's like, if you get into it over here.

Lee laughed and then reminded me that even though this was a rather modern couple, of German descent, they remembered from their background the words to release this man from the spell. He added that Saint John the Baptist is a powerful spirit in Hex and in Voodoo.

JM: You said in the *Sandlapper* article that you were drawn to this place, that you felt you'd lived here before.

LG: Oh, yes, I lived once in Charleston and twice here in the county.

JM: Is that a common belief around here?

I asked this, knowing the rather conservative Protestant backgrounds of most of the people.

LG: I don't know how common it is, because you don't talk about these things very much. But this boy, who is such a good Hex, believes he's been here before and was even my nephew during the Civil War.

JM: Were you drawn to this particular house?

LG: This house is a Hex house. It was built by a Hex.

JM: How do you know that?

LG: Partly by the orientation, partly by the administration, and partly by the holly trees.

JM: Do holly trees have some special meaning? There were several large holly trees in the front yard.

LG: Oh, yes. For one thing, the holly tree is supposed to keep evil spirits away. And hollies protect a house from lightning and from being burned. This house was here during the Civil War, and all the other ones around here were burned during Sherman's march to the sea. Only this one was hardly touched. This house is oriented with the earth. It faces directly west and anyone coming toward it must face east. If you ever get into the Masonic orders, you'll find that advancing toward the east is very important. To approach this house you must face the rising sun, something an evil spirit would not want to do. The important part of it is that this house is built on the highest point of land between two bodies of moving water. There's 13 Mile Creek, which you crossed to get here, and the Saluda River. It also has three front doors, so you are able to enter physically, emotionally, and spiritually.

JM: Do you know who owned the house before?

He nodded and proceeded to tell me that the house had belonged to a number of families over the years, most recently the family of Frau Ingleman, one of the women who were burned as a witch in Fairfield County.

JM: Now you got me, I did not know there were women burned as witches in South Carolina.

LG: Not burned to death. . . . They were hanged by their hands and the soles of their feet were burned off. Have you not read my article called "The Witches of Fairfield," which was published in *Fate* magazine? Here, I'll show some of it to you, although this is not the full account.

He fumbled through his papers and produced a notebook, which he handed to me.

LG: I keep a lot of my notes on magic in this.

JM: What is this language?

I was unable to decipher the hieroglyphs I saw before me. I later learned in E. A. Wallis Budge's tome, *Amulets and Superstitions,* that this script is called Theban Script. It is Greek in origin and "is said to have been invented by Honorius, a Theban, and to have been handed down by Peter of Apono" (403). It is now commonly called "The Witches Alphabet," according to the *Encyclopedia of Wicca and Witchcraft,* by Raven Grimassi, and has been employed by a variety of occult groups from the 16th century onward.

LG: I suppose you'd call them witches' runes. Been used for years to keep things secret. Let me read you from a transcript. It was supposed to have been part of a history of Fairfield County.

Lee then read to me the transcript of the handwritten account of the trial and persecution of accused witches in late 18th-century South Carolina. A copy of the original document is available in microfilm in the Lyman C. Draper Manuscript Collection at the South Carolina Department of Archives and History, located in Columbia, South Carolina.

The ellipses and dashes in the excerpt below indicate illegible or gaps in the text. The parenthetical numbers indicate the page number of the original manuscript copy from the microfilm. Readers will note that the transcript reflects the educational level of the writer and the changes that have occurred in the common spelling of English words and changes in accepted grammar.

There had always been witches and wizards in Fairfield (4). In the old time they were comparatively harmless. They may have sailed through the air on brooms, or braided the necks of the horses at night. All believed in them, but few suffered from them. But in 1782, they became spiteful and mischievous, damaging the cattle of a fearful rate, oppressing hysterical women, and riding★ stout men to their great annoyance and discomfort. Too far did they go in their . . . practices that they could no longer wel-

---

★This phrase refers to a supposed supernatural act of a spirit attacking and molesting a person in their sleep. The practice is commonly known as "hag-riding." In modern times, this is thought by the scientific community to be the result of sleep apnea.

come with, and the people (that is one in twenty) concluded to arrest them in their evil doings, and bring them, or some of them, to . . . punishment (5). The parties accused were old man . . . and his wife, Sally Smith, and the dreadful old Mary Ingleman. The three first had laid evil hands on Rosy Henley and her sister and damaged many cattle in the Eastern quarter of the county. Rosy was much more tormented than her sister, but both were greatly troubled. Lying in her bed, she could not be prevented, by the utmost exertions of four strong men, from rising up, and clinging to the ceiling; they were both bitten on the neck and shoulders, and struck over with pins and splinters (6). Their case was dreadful. The testimony was duly made out, well authenticated and forwarded to the Bench of Witch Doctors appointed to preside over the witch trial, which was held at Manor Hills, 5 miles . . . from the county capital. The testimony against the arch offender, Mary Ingleman, was ample and voluminous, for much of it was taken down in writing (7). Adam Free testified against his mother, when she asked him for a cow, and he refused, it shortly after sprang up with a convulsive bound, fell, and broke its neck. And that sometimes his cattle gave blood instead of milk. Jacob ———, the grandson of the prisoner, testified that on one occasion his grandmother turned him into a horse and rode him six miles to Major Pearson's apple orchard on Broad river. Whilst she was filling her bag with apples, his eye was attracted by the beautiful red apples that hung over him (8). He put up his long horse head to obtain a stealthy supply, and whilst attempting to do so, she drove a punch into his cheek, from the effects of which he did not soon recover. Martha Holly, alias ——— Haw, testified that Mrs. Ingleman had greatly afflicted her. She put up balls of hair with pins sticking out, way all over the neck and shoulders stuck full of pins and splinters, and deprived of all peace and comfort.

The chief witness was Isaac Collins. He testified that on one occasion he took his trusty rifle and went out on a deer hunt around Noe Tyres' old field (9). He saw a deer and . . . at it several times . . . with unavailing efforts to procure venison, he drew his ball, split it open, and inserted in it a thin sliver of silver ramming down his ball. So improved, he raised up his piece and fired. Instead of a deer, a black cat with its fore leg shivered, hopped off before him. Such is the mighty power of the . . . metal. In a day or two, Isaac was engaged in plowing corn. In the heat of the day, he . . . to a delightful spring of water near the cornfield

(10). When he arrived at the spring, he found Mrs. Ingleman seated near it with her arm in a sling. Collins inquired how she was, and the old witch replied "Well, but for an injury to my arm." She held it up as best she could, and said to Collins, "This is your work." So it turned out that Mrs. Ingleman was the deer, the black cat and again herself! Isaac testified further that Mrs. Ingleman turned him into a horse, and rode him to a grand witch convention. On the way the Devil rode up by her side and observed, "Mother Ingleman, you have a splendid horse." (11). "Shhhh," said she, "This is that rascal Collins." He said the witch convention was a splendid affair. He never could locate the place of meeting, but supposed it somewhere in North America.

The evidence was held more than sufficient. The accused could offer nothing in their defense and were all convicted. According to the sentence, they were ... tied up to the joists of the shanty in which they were tried, whipped and then placed with their feet to a bark fire, and confined there until the soles popped off (12). Such was the result of this miserable trial.

Sally Smith faced worse than the other convicts, for after receiving her flogging and burning, in attempting to hobble home, she was overtaken by a party, who cast her down, and placed a pine log across her neck. She could not stir, and the next day was relieved by a benevolent person passing along the path.

As Lee finished reading this account, he looked up at me and burst out laughing, "You are sitting there looking totally incredulous! You get into something when you deal with this life! This is where magic gets real!"

Author's note: Apparently, Mrs. Ingleman became the victim of a typical witch persecution with charges of milk stealing and cow molestation, hag riding, attending witches' sabbaths, rolling witch's balls and so forth. Such signs were typical of charges filed by people of German and Appalachian origin. It is interesting to note that the "trial" of Mrs. Ingleman and the other defendants was not held before a conventional court of law but by "a bench of Witch Doctors," according to Theresa M. Hicks in the section "Did you hear about . . . Witchcraft in South Carolina?" found on the website, Believe it or not? South Carolina Heresies, Folklore, Shocking Revelations, Murder, Mayhem & Mystery. Hicks points out that accusations of and trials for witchcraft continued into the first quarter of the 19th century: "In 1825, Barbara Powers was accused of turning a girl into a horse and rode her to Cheraw. This case went on appeal and became well-known. The case of Mary Ingleman was settled in the lower court and is less well-known." (par. 5).

CHAPTER SIX

Interview
Powwow–Hexerei: An Eclectic Practice

I would rather have a mind opened by wonder than one closed by belief.
—Gerry Spence, *How to Argue and Win Every Time*

Either magic works or it doesn't. I don't worry too much about the theory.
—Lee Raus Gandee, Hexenmeister

Adventures in Powwow Healing

As I continued interviewing Lee Gandee, I began to learn and practice some of the healing techniques he taught me. A couple of instances occurred that made me turn to these remedies, as the usual treatments were not immediately available. One day, my lit cigarette broke as I attempted to flick the ash out the car window. I pulled the car over and stopped, realizing I had a second-degree burn between my first two fingers. Of course, I was in the car and did not have any healing salve available. I remembered the incantation for burns from John George Hohman's *The Long Lost Friend* (see Appendix). I spoke the words quickly over the burn, with, frankly, no expectation of success. I was stunned when the pain immediately subsided and the redness disappeared within a minute. I sat there in amazement and rubbed the area, sure I would still feel pain.

Two days later, while trying to repair my mother's radio, I dropped a soldering iron across the top of my fingers of my left hand. I heard the crackle and smelled the burning skin before I felt the pain. No one was home, and I was in agony. I once again resorted to the incantation for burns. Once again, the pain was gone within seconds. Although some redness remained for a few days, this considerable burn healed quickly, leaving only a small scar.

I could hardly wait until the next week, when I could share my experiences with Lee.

When I told him about this episode, Lee asked, "Which one did you use?"

Lee was, of course, referring to the incantations in *The Long Lost Friend*. Lee did not personally use Hohman extensively. With his developed ability to project psychic energy, he really did not need the formal incantation as a vehicle though he considered it useful and would occasionally quote from it. He told me that he had once seen a copy in the original German, dating from the mid-19th century. The copy belonged to a local Dutch Fork family, and it was a treasured heirloom.

"'The one that begins "Burn, I blow on thee. . . ."'" I replied. "I did just as the book indicated: 'It [the breath] must be blown on three times in the same breath, like the fire by the sun.' You indicated that when you cured the burns on your arms, you used a mirror. Was that really necessary?

Lee replied, "I don't think so. I just wanted to see what I was doing. . . . I thought maybe looking at the image would help, 'cause normally you would look at the person you're working for; if he's around." (See Chapter Four: Lee Gandee: Hexenmeister, Teacher, Friend, where we discuss his ability to heal at a distance.)

"I was wondering if mirrors play a role, a part, in Hexerei," I said.

"Well, there are some [uses]. . . ." Lee began. "There is the ceremony of the 'Dead Man's Mirror.' You have to have a dead man's mirror to work it. . . . You scry into a dead man's mirror. . . . I did this for an old couple on the other side of Lexington [South Carolina]."

"Was that for the young boy?" I asked. "I've been reading that a lot of people use not only mirrors but water to scry."

I was referring to an account of Lee's attempting to locate a missing son for an old couple. They had lost touch with their oldest son many years before. The ritual apparently allowed a younger sibling to have vision of deceased relatives and his brother and to deduce that the older boy had met with ill fortune. The elder brother was imprisoned in another state. Apparently, this gave the old couple enough information to eventually locate their missing son and even visit him in prison.

"Oh, yes, that's what they use with the dead man's mirror," Lee explained. "You hold the mirror in your hand in front of you, and you have the water in a glass jar or jug on a table behind your left shoulder. You hold a the mirror so that you can see a flame or lamp on the other side of the jug of water so that it looks like the flame or light is inside the jug of water. . . . You look in the mirror. . . . I couldn't see anything but the pyrotechnics in the water and neither could the old couple, but this boy looked in and started seeing pictures almost as soon as he went into trance. He saw his father and grandfather at work, right there on the place where they lived. He told that he saw his great grandfather who had a deformed, broken hand that was bent back like this (toward the wrist). . . . [He] really impressed the old couple with the things he saw."

"Why do you think the young boy could see the images when no one else could?"

"I don't know, maybe the rest of us did not go into trance. I guess that was it. But I've found that you can scry in a glass of water as easily as with all that rigmarole," Lee said.

I then recounted a story of a teenaged friend's mother who used a brass bowl filled with water to deduce the activities of her truck driver husband while he was out on the road.

"She claimed to have learned of his infidelities. . . . 'Course, I don't know about her mental stability. . . . She was known to be a little off."

"Well, if you get the reputation of doing things like that, you get that reputation whether you are or not. Then you say, 'Oh, I saw in a glass of water that you were in Selma, Alabama night before last with Kiki or who-ever. . . . We're going to get a divorce right away if that keeps up. . . .' Well, if you haven't been [fooling around] then you've been taken advantage of by a glass of water . . . and you do end up thinking the person is a little off," Lee remarked.

"I was wondering about the trance state?"

"Well, about the best way I can make out, the best way to explain it is the way Seth does, in his book on the nature of personal reality. Our thoughts, emotions and beliefs have a physical reality and when properly focused, can give your mind the ability to do incredible things. This is what Hex is all about!" Lee exclaimed.

Lee was referring to the phenomenon of Seth, a discarnate entity chan-neled through Jane Roberts. Roberts wrote summaries of her trance-state communications from Seth, which totaled 10 volumes before her death in

1984. *The Seth Material* summarized the channeled messages from Seth to Roberts from 1963-1969; beginning in 1970, the Seth entity dictated information directly, which Roberts transcribed into several other volumes.

Then Lee changed the subject and began to recount a story from the night before, when he had a strange phone call. Here's how Lee told me about it:

"I mean to say I had a surprise last night! I was astounded, 'cause a girl called me up and said, 'I'm Cindy M———. Do you remember me?'"

"I can't place you," I said.

"I'm Dick's girlfriend. . . ." she said.

And I knew Dick, or thought I knew him pretty well. "Well, how are you doing?" I said.

"I'm not doing too well right now."

"How's Dick?" I said.

"Oh, he's in a terrible state. That's why I called you. . . . I want to find out if we can bring him over'"

And I said, "What happened?"

"Oh!" she said. "He tore the apartment completely to pieces, and broke my nose——"

"Maybe you should turn that thing off," Lee said to me, referring to the tape recorder.

"I won't use any names," I replied.

So, Lee resumed his story. . . .

So, I said, "Bring him on, and I'll do what I can for him."

When they got there with another individual, a friend who came along to protect her from Dick, I suppose. Anyway, when Dick came in I was shocked. If I ever saw someone who was possessed by an evil spirit, he had to be. . . . And he was just as belligerent as could be, almost insanely preoccupied with himself. I had him sit down, and he wanted me to challenge the evil spirit by the power of the God that I believed in, and he would defend himself by the power of Satan and so on. . . . I didn't raise my voice, didn't do anything, because, in a case like that, the only thing to do is to just use sweet patience and reason. I told him that there wasn't any challenge as I could see, because good and evil didn't exist except in the mind of the person, and it was for him to decide which one he wanted in there with him. That kept on for about an hour, with this other self just violent, just trying to assert itself—it's s right over this friend of mine—to do anything with him it pleased. I kept saying that it was Dick's decision, but that nobody had any devils in them except the ones they'd created themselves. I told him if he preferred to believe that there was a devil in him that was his business but, as far as I was concerned, I was not worried at all because I didn't believe in the existence of devils with their own existence. And so, on it went, until finally, it just gave up, I think.... Dick turned back into Dick and looked at the girl like he was just completely strange....

Dick couldn't figure out what had happened and looked at my bottle collection and looked at his hands all covered in blood and said "I'm burning up inside, can I go get some water?" He went in the kitchen and washed his hands, drank some water, looked at his girlfriend and said "Did I do that?"

"Yes you did!" she said, and at that he became very tender, very affectionate, apologized, kissed her and everything seemed all right.

"What do you think was actually happening?" I asked.

"Well, I don't know what to think about it! Whether he would say today that it never happened or what happened, or could even tell you what happened.... Anyway, they left and took her to a doctor and then went to clean up the apartment but, I just don't know.... What a shameful state he was in...."

"That's really interesting," I said. "You know, in the Eastern religions, they maintain that man creates his own devils, his own hells and his own heavens."

"Oh, I believe that! Christianity teaches that, the church doesn't, but Christianity does, because Jesus said, 'the Kingdom of heaven is within you.' That's the same as saying that you have to create it there, because whatever you do is what you put there. Most people go through life believing that life happens to them, but in fact, they created it themselves."

"That experience with Dick must have been an unnerving experience," I commented.

"Well, this entity claimed to the last that it was Lucifer and I don't hold myself worthy of visitations by spirits of that rank even if they are fallen spirits. I don't know.... Makes me wonder about the man's stability a little bit, because I can imagine a discarnate spirit taking over somebody, yes, in fact it's awful.... The insane asylum is full of people who've had such spirits take them over, but they don't go around saying they're Lucifer unless they're in the same shape as people who go around saying they're Napoleon or somebody. I just know that boy too well, and he's a bad boy, but he's no Lucifer," Lee laughed.

"But he had created—"

Lee interrupted me. "I don't know if it was just ego trying to find some way out because he has a bad situation with himself: out of work, a highly intelligent person. He's an orphan, has no one that he's close to except this Mary and he is a witch, but not a Hexenmeister. He's, what do you call it, a coven master and his coven had deserted him. He thought that the coven was what put him in this shape, after it was over. . . . that they were conspiring against him. I said, 'Well, it's up to you how much power you give them. They have as much power over you as you think they have. If you want to, set them up and make it easy for them to do something to you. If not, just ignore it.' So, he seems to be pretty well straightened out. He took my pentagram from off the wall, and he called it a Star of David. (*Author's note:* A pentagram is *not* a Star of David. A pentagram has five points. A Star of David has six.) I explained the symbolism to him and told him it had kept Israel safe for 2000 years, so it would protect him against the influence of his witch buddies in the coven. I told him all he had to do was to look at the stability of the pyramid and hold on to that stability and let the other instability take care of itself. I think he saw the stability, and he'll be all right for a little while. Maybe when he gets a job or something, he'll be okay."

"Using" to Heal: Lee Does a Healing on Me

During our time together Lee performed several healings on me.

The first healing Lee performed on me was about two months after I met him. Shortly after I arrived that Wednesday morning, we were discussing the Vietnam War, and I unconsciously started rubbing my jaw. When I was younger and under stress, I used to grind my teeth in my sleep, which would leave my jaw aching and sore.

Lee noticed this and asked me what was wrong.

"Oh, my jaw is aching from bruxing my teeth while I'm sleeping. I don't suppose you could fix it for me?"

"Are you asking me?"

"I guess so!" I said, thinking that otherwise I was stuck with the pain for the rest of the day.

"All right," he said, as he rose from his chair and cupped his hands on either side of my face.

"Oh, brother!" I thought, as he began to chant. I'd tried to help myself before with massage and medication, with little success.

All of a sudden, I noticed the warmth of his hands and a tingling in the part of my jaw where the bones met. I kept very still for what seemed only about a minute. As he took his hands away and returned to his chair, I noticed that the dull, hard ache in my jaw was gone.

The look of amazement on my face betrayed my thoughts, because Lee looked at me, chuckled and said, "You think this is all some trick of the mind! Doesn't hurt anymore, does it?"

"I'm sorry Lee, I don't mean to seem ungrateful, I'm just surprised. This is really amazing! Thank you very much!"

"You're welcome," he said. "If you hang around here, you'll get used to this sort of thing."

The next time Lee did a healing on me was early one morning, when I arrived at his house with a large bruise on my right forearm. I had carelessly walked into a raised counter-top. Like my mother, when I bump into something, the bruise quickly blackens and spreads, leaving a large, painful, ugly-looking area. Lee spotted it as I sat down and asked me about it as I turned on my tape recorder.

"Does it hurt?" Lee asked.

"Just a bit," I replied. "Think you could fix it?"

"Can I see it for a second?"

"Sure," I said and extended my arm to him. He held it gently in his left hand and fixed his gaze on the bruise. With his right hand, he formed a fist with the thumb extended and pointing downward. As he slowly circled the bruise counterclockwise, I could hear him whispering a famous chant for bruises:

> Bruise, thou shalt not heat;
> Bruise, thou shalt not sweat;
> Bruise, thou shalt not run,
> No-more than Virgin Mary shall bring forth another son.

He then made the sign of the cross three times

I must admit, I felt a tingling sensation in the area of the bruise. He finished by making the sign of the cross with his thumb pointed downward. He looked up and smiled at me.

"It should feel better soon."

"Okay, thanks!" I replied.

As I sat down, I remember thinking to myself, "Anything will be an improvement on what I have now." As our conversation drifted to other things, I forgot the bruise for about twenty minutes. Suddenly I remembered and glanced quickly at my arm. To my shock, the bruise was totally gone and so was the aching. It was as if I had never been injured at all. I held up my arm to him and said, "Hey, look at my arm!"

"Feel better?" he asked.

"The bruise is completely gone!" I exclaimed.

"Uh-huh," he said, as he lit his pipe. "What did you expect?"

"I don't know! Thanks!"

"Don't mention it!" Lee said.

It was like that with Lee. The miraculous became so commonplace that those around him just got used to it. As for Lee, he was totally casual in his manner and response, as if he had done nothing more than open a window.

On another occasion, I was telling Lee about "using" for a painful, inflamed scratch on my girlfriend's leg. As we watched, it stopped bleeding and the inflammation subsided, leaving only a small white scar.

"One of the things that fascinates me about 'using' is how I was able to be effective upon my girlfriend's leg. She wasn't even aware I was doing it; she was absorbed in television while I was doing the ritual. How do you explain it?"

Lee replied, "How do you explain it? How do you explain the fact that when the cows' horns are sawed off, with all the copious bleeding on each side of their heads, but when my grandmother said the words to stop bleeding and the bleeding would stop? How did Mike heal the dog who had been run over? Did he have to tell the dog? How do the cows know it?"

"But in Beaufort, they [the root doctors] base everything on the fact that you must know you're being worked upon." I said.

"That's Voodoo. There's things a lot more subtle than Voodoo," Lee said.

"I agree, I saw it work," I said, referring to the incident with the inflamed scratch on my girlfriend's leg.

"I don't know if I've ever been able to explain it to myself," he continued. "If you can understand what this man is saying in this book, you will have the practice of magic figured out!" he said, rising from his chair, retrieving a book and handing it to me.

"Huna magic!" I remarked, looking at the text. "I'd like to read this."

"It's a classic," Lee replied. "He [the author] spent 40 years in Hawaii trying to find out the secrets of Kahuna [traditional Hawaiian healers] magic. He accepted their theories on how it worked. I really don't know that I accept their theories, that there are tangible things that connect humans together, but I don't know that I don't believe it. I use it just as if it were true, and I find that it works just the same, if it is true or not. Either magic works or it doesn't. I don't worry too much about the theory," Lee said with a chuckle.

We now moved to another topic of how mental energy is transmitted from a Powwow to a person or an animal and the difference between the practice of hypnotism and a magical process called magnetism.

"In your book," I began, "you used the name Cuz, the hypnotist. I was told by my psychology professor, who is a hypnotist, that it [hypnotism] is a very dangerous thing if you don't know exactly what you're doing, yet you seem to have had no trouble with it."

"Well, he'd read a book that said that somewhere," Lee replied.

"Had you studied hypnotism?"

"No. I got out an old book that was written before the Civil War, and people back then didn't know how dangerous it was," he said, smiling, "so they didn't worry about it. Since then I have found out that practically everybody—even the people around here [the Dutch Fork area—were up to their eyes in hypnotism back then, calling it 'animal magnetism' and [they] were 'magnetizing' one another. I magnetized Cuz [from the book]. I thought I was hypnotizing him, but I was actually magnetizing him."

"What's the difference?" I asked.

"Oh, there's one hell of a difference!" he replied. "Because if you magnetize somebody, you are doing exactly what these Kahunas are doing with their *akka* substance [psychic energy]. You are just impregnating and permeating a person with your own substance. All of these commands and things go right through these little lines that he [the author] is talking about; directly into the person, and the person the person doesn't have to be told audibly what to do. You can just will what he does, and he does it 'cause you are connected by the energy trail you have established with that person either by mental projection or physical touch."

Lee went on to talk about how, in Russia, certain college researchers are trying to establish the existence of and use this connection between all living things.

"What's the status on the 'ether' in modern science?" Lee asked.

"It is not used anymore" I replied.

Lee went on to say that several authors have postulated that one need not actually touch a person, place or thing to establish a contact or a channel through which to move energy. You can even follow the connection they have made with another individual and apparently transmit elements of your own conscious energy down that channel.

I was recently asked to visit a dear friend's mother who had lapsed into a coma in Pennsylvania. In a trance state, I was able to follow my connection with him and then connect to his connection with his mother, which was very strong, since he had recently visited her in the hospital. I was asked to examine her current condition and to try to bring her words of peace and comfort. This took a tremendous psychic effort on my part, but I was able to describe her appearance and the hospital room in detail and relay his mother's unspoken needs to him. This person is also a powerful Powwow and was able with that information, to offer his mother great emotional and spiritual comfort during her last days. He and his wife are both wonderful examples of the modern Powwow tradition.

The Mind Is a Powerful Thing

To illustrate his point about the mind's ability to affect the physical body, Lee referred to [pioneering hypnotist] Phineas Parkhurst Quimby (1802-1866). Quimby had a famous case: A woman was brought to him, dying from edema. As Quimby pursued the initial investigation, he learned that the woman had experienced the loss of a loved one, who drowned after a quarrel. Now, consumed with guilt and regret, she was, in effect, unconsciously drowning herself in her own body fluids. Quimby hypnotized her and found out about the loved one drowning and the guilt and was able to reverse the woman's condition and thereby facilitate her partial recovery.

Lee then spoke of the history of this idea of psychic manifestation in the popular culture of the 18th and 19th century. Psychic manifestation was based on the belief that someone's mental state influences their physical and perceptional reality and, even unconsciously, manifests in their life's events. Even if someone became sick, injured or died, these events were sometimes traceable to the individual's belief in the impact of their past transgressions. On the other hand, if someone experienced good health or wealth, this was traceable to their positive relationship with others and their overall positive mental state. A person's relationship with the Divine also affected their overall state of physical and mental health. It was a common belief that good fortune and material prosperity was a sign of Divine approval.

"Isn't it convenient? Now you really don't have to worry over the misfortunes of others. After all, they brought it on themselves," Lee said, only half-jokingly.

Some ideas really seem to endure over the centuries: A tragic modern manifestation of this idea is that diseases like AIDS are, in fact, an expression of Divine disapproval. This rather sophisticated form of mind control, Lee asserted, combined with a large dose of guilt, will easily take on a physical manifestation.

I asked Lee if he thought this ability to manifest guilt was more common in women.

"Oh, it does in men, too," he quickly responded. "So one of the things I like about my system [Hexerei] is that I just don't deal in guilt. In the first place, in Hexerei, we don't have any rules to follow except one, and it's supposed to be the one the witches follow 'If it hurts nobody, do what you please.' If you think about it," he added, "it's pretty restrictive! On the other hand, there are things you can do that don't hurt anybody, but that our society, our culture, our religion just prohibit for the sake of prohibiting. A classic example of it would be many of the ideas surrounding sex. As long as it doesn't contaminate somebody with disease or cause and unwanted pregnancy, I believe anybody ought to be able to have sex with anybody they choose."

During the time I knew Lee, he struggled with, and eventually embraced, his own homosexuality. As many who have read Lee's book know, he devotes no small part of it to his struggles with and coming to understand his homosexuality. Like many people his age, he had attempted for many years to lead a straight, heterosexual life but found himself increasingly trapped by his feelings on one side and his social persona on the other. I believe his memories of an earlier life as a female in ancient Minos was a psychic manifestation of his inner struggle and a way in which he could rationalize, cope and express his newly realized sexual identity in a positive manner. I never shared this insight with Lee. His sexuality was not my concern or my interest beyond how it affected his practice of Powwow.

In many ways, his book, *Strange Experience: Secrets of a Hexenmeister*, was an attempt to "come out" in the context of telling the story of his interest in Hexerei. The book jockeys back and forth between these two parts of his personal history. Its publication was, according to Lee, devastating to his immediate family, leaving him further estranged from his wife. The local community, at that time very small, shuddered at the revelation. In the years that I knew Lee, I heard him express regret for the hurt his revelation had caused, but never for having done it. To remain closeted and living a lie would have been too much for him to personally bear.

Was Lee a Real Shaman?

During the writing of this manuscript, a friend, after reading parts of this manuscript, asked me if I thought Lee was really a shaman or simply a community healer like the charmers of the British Isles. The answer, I believe, is to be found in the writings of the famous scholar of religions, Mircea Eliade. Eliade considered the practice of shamanism to be one of purposefully altering one's awareness; to be able to transcend the normal state of awareness to achieve some personal or spiritual objective. In this sense, shamanism is properly termed a practice rather than a religion, although the practice may be undertaken for religious purposes. Eliade referred to this practice as:

. . . the passage from one cosmic region to another—from earth to sky or from earth to the underworld. The shaman knows the mystery of the breakthrough in plane. This communication among the cosmic zones is made possible by the very structure of the universe." (259)

Given this definition, Lee Gandee incorporated travel to other realms by altering his consciousness to locate people or information. Like the Siberian shamans of the Tungus people, referred to by Eliade, Lee would place himself in a trance state in order to perform a task at the request of others, or for his own needs. To perform a healing, one must enter a state of trance so the presence of the Divine can move through the healer to the healed.

Also like the Tungus shaman, Lee was brought to this practice through a series of incidents in his life that acted as an initiation. His family history, cultural beliefs and practice acted as a catalyst for what manifested in his adolescence and later life.

In studying the life histories of Hindu holy men, both historical and hagiographic, these elements of shamanic initiation and practice present themselves in much the same way in a non-western culture. The common theme or scenario is of a normal child, who upon experiencing a traumatic event, whether physical, emotional or social, breaks from his former life and begins to pursue a spiritual path. An example of this transformation would be the death-like experience of the boy who was to become Ramana Maharishi, the great spiritual teacher of South India.

Common manifestations of spiritual growth or *siddhis,* as they are called in the Hindu tradition, include trance states resulting in Divine communication. Such a state was manifested by the great 19th-century Bengali sage, Ramakrishna Paramahamsa. Other siddhis include physical bi-location of consciousness, as was manifested by the mystic, Shridi Sai Baba, and the ability to heal emotional and physical illness, as was manifested by the great exponent of Advaita Vedanta, Adi Shankara. All of these practices and many others are shamanic in method and expression.

While I am not about to claim that Lee or the other people featured in this book have a spiritual parity with the above-mentioned Hindu holy men, they, like the shamans or healers in this book, all manifest some of the characteristics and engage in similar practices as monks, sadhus, and saints across the world. All shamans, healers, and saintly people tend to behave in shaman-like ways. As Eliade said, they "have played an essential role in the defense of the psychic integrity of the community" (508). These American shamans, like their Eastern counterparts, live at the edge of society. They are engaged yet removed from the cultural ebb and flow.

CHAPTER SEVEN

The World of the Unseen

I am too much of a skeptic to deny the possibility of anything.

—Thomas Henry Huxley (1825–1895)

The whole problem with the world is that fools and fanatics are always so certain of themselves, but wiser people so full of doubts.

—Bertrand Russell, (1872–1970)

JUNE 1975

I made the next phone call to Lee early one lovely summer day.

"Good morning, Lee. Would it be all right if I stopped by today?"

"Sure," he replied, "come right on out, there's somewhere I want us to go."

"Will we need to take my car?" I asked, knowing Lee did not have access to a car until his wife returned from work.

"No, nothing like that! You'll see."

When I arrived, he was sitting in his room smoking his pipe as usual. I thanked him for his time and brought him the pipe cleaners he'd asked for earlier. I always tried to compensate him for his time in some small way.

I began this session by asking, "You were talking last time about the fact that miracles are not supported by the religious establishment; can you elaborate on that? Why would the church be against miracles?"

It's simple," Lee replied. "Because they cannot control the message of the miracle or the people who produce them. The Western church has never been kind to those who make their own connections to the almighty. Mystics, healers and witches have always found themselves at odds with the religious establishment because they operate outside the realm of doctrine. Also, without knowing it, they have gradually bought into the scientific rational view of reality hook, line and sinker."

"But why?" I asked. "Most religions base their doctrines on some from of mystical experience."

"Absolutely!" He laughed. "Then the religious establishment codifies and analyzes it and rewrites it to make it say what they wish it to say and condemns you if you question them. It's all about control, but it also goes deeper than that.

"The Hindus you were talking about last time believe that god is the very base of your being, your innermost self and your essence. Most people in the West think of god as a political entity, like a great cosmic monarch, a courtroom judge, the universal policeman who makes and enforces the laws he supposedly made and of course, the church as his official bureaucracy and representative. The idea that god could be present in every human being or in the natural world defies the idea of this universal king and the sense of justice. It becomes socially preposterous for an individual to claim that he has an identity with or some direct knowledge of this king of the universe and therefore the mystical experience, in those terms is subversive. See what I mean?" Lee concluded.

"I think so." I thought for a moment. "So, if I have a mystical experience and have a oneness with the divine, I must be crazy or subversive, because that flies in the face of tradition and makes the spiritual authorities irrelevant."

"That's it exactly!" he said, with a hearty laugh, and added, "So if you find god, you'd better keep it to yourself. Sort of like seeing a ghost or a UFO, if you tell anyone, they'll put you in the booby hatch!"

We both laughed heartily.

"Many mystics in the past have found themselves considered heretics, which in the old days was a very serious charge that could get you burned at the stake," Lee said soberly. "Yes, but what about guys like St. John of the Cross?" I asked. "I was just reading about him for a class and he had some pretty intense mystical experiences." I had been studying *The Dark Night of the Soul* in a class on apocalyptic literature.

Lee replied, "Sure, but if you read closely, you'll see he's careful to keep himself and god in two different spheres. No religious authority is going to tolerate religious insubordination of that type. Nothing could be worse for religious authority than a wave of mystical experiences. Look at the stigmatic who physically manifests the wounds of Christ. They are usually kept away from public view especially if they happen to be priests or nuns."

I was stunned. "Seriously, you mean people do this in this day and age?" I had not, at that time heard of the phenomena of stigmata.

"See how conditioned you are to expect only that which society tells you is reality? Like I just said, God, in the Western mind, is constructed on the model of a medieval king, and seated upon his throne in heaven, jealously guarding his kingdom from hostile forces, like the devil, and dispensing justice to his human subjects. Anything that goes against his authority or the authority of his representatives on earth must be considered as hostile. Have you ever looked at a church and the way it's built? It's set up like a throne room with everyone kneeling in submission before the throne. Kneeling before the king was established because it made you less able to launch a sudden attack. Have you ever noticed that in church ritual the supplicant treats god like a monarch by flattering him with phrases like 'King of Kings, Lord of Lords, ruler of all' and so forth?"

"I never thought of it that way," I said, "but I see your point. Why would the church structure it like that?"

"It was all they knew at the time. You must remember from your history of western civilization class that as the Roman idea of the Divine ruler declined in the late empire, as the emperors became less effective and downright crazy at times, the religious administration behind the throne was searching for a new king they could get behind, one that would not become decadent or insane, and one whose political and spiritual authority and power could not be questioned. If I were going to administrate for a king, wouldn't you want one like that? Anyway, the Roman church found such a king in Jesus and since he was, by that time, the stuff of legend, he could not embarrass them, and they could make him say what they wanted him to say to suit their needs." Lee concluded.

"I have to ask this, Lee. Do you believe in God?"

"Of course! That should be obvious. What made you ask that question?" Lee looked at me curiously.

"I don't know. I guess that you were talking about how it was all energy, that we are all energy. . . . How you go into a church and all the confusing energy. . . ." I trailed off, clearly feeling a bit overwhelmed by this conversation.

"That does not change the idea of God, Jack. It just expands it. God has two aspects; personal and impersonal, just like you do."

"I don't understand."

"No, you probably don't right now. Let me put it this way. There is a conscious entity that comprises the entire universe and yet is beyond it. It has always been just as it is. Out of that energy comes a will to experience, a will to observe. The most common idea of God comes out of a second level of will to experience, which in turn must create objects like the world, and you and me to have that experience. God, in an anthropomorphic sense, like Jesus, like Jehovah, or other Gods with forms and names, are composites created by us out of our awareness of its presence and our own experience. We evolved out of that Divine will, that desire to exist and create God's form, in a kind of circular process."

"Does that mean that these Gods with name and form really don't exist?"

"Absolutely not! God is very real. You know from your science classes that energy can't be created or destroyed, only moved, concentrated and contained, like in a battery. The God you know and pray to is like that battery, and it gets recharged by your worship and devotion, which send energy to it. This form of God needs your love and prayers, so he answers them. He comes when you need him and meets your need and helps you grow spiritually. It is a reciprocal relationship on a cosmic scale, but it means that God is very real. See what I mean?"

"I guess!" I said, trying to absorb this new cosmic view of the Divine. "So the God we call Jesus after 1,975 years of devotion and worship would be very powerful!"

"Exactly, why else should we call on him when we do a healing and it works! It's because he does respond in that form and to that name. We are just a wire through which the connection is made. That connection goes all the way back to the source of everything and then back again. We are just consciously tapping into it for a split second. The dimension of spirit entities is just another point of connection. The circuit is complete at every moment all the time in one continuous flow. That is why Jesus says

'I am in the father and you are in me.' He understood that connection."

"Would that mean if no one worshipped Jesus he would disappear?" I asked.

"No," he replied, laughing. "He would just adopt another form that we did worship. God has done this countless times and appears to other people in a form they can recognize and respond to. How do you think there got to be so many gods? This is why we can never be separate from God, except in our delusions that we somehow are different. Without that divine energy, we would not exist."

"That sounds a bit like some of the Eastern religions."

"I suppose so. Ask yourself, why would God create an entire universe and then decide to show himself only to a tiny section of it? Why would such a being then decide that one tiny group of his creation were the only ones he really cared about? How utterly stupid! That whole idea is our minds, trying to contain God, put him a box that looks like us, sounds like us, so we can think we've got it all figured out. Even worse, to supposedly give us a reason for separating ourselves from one another; from being unkind to each other, fighting over whose god is better or loves them more! How very human such a god would be: insecure, jealous, greedy and petty. Sounds pretty human to me! Sort of like the ancient Greeks and Romans whose gods were just like them, only more powerful."

"I understand. It is very hard for humans to think in abstract terms like energies, and they need to give god a name. That's why we have so many images and names for God!" I could see the connections now, and it was really exciting to hear Lee's perspective.

"Exactly, it's why those who wield power over the religious establishment are afraid of mystics and witches and those who might let the cat out of the bag and cause chaos."

"Okay, but what role does the church and conventional religion play in all this?" This was the part that was getting confusing to me.

Lee said, "Religions and churches are an attempt to set forth some structure and authority and control over this mystical form of human awareness. It all breaks down to one word: control!"

"But what does that have to do with Hexerei?" I felt like we were getting way off the subject.

"It has everything to do with it. The point is that most mystical traditions that lead you to some form of direct contact with the divine are going to be seen, on occasion, as at odds with the religious powers that be. Therefore, traditions like Hexerei have always had to live outside society. You remember reading about the Inquisition? What do you think that was all about? Authority and control, that's what it was all about! The church had to try to get out and stamp out all the remnants of the old indigenous European religions and anything that might reduce people's dependence on the church. Most of the thousands of people tortured and killed were women who practiced some from of mystical or herbal healing, divination, or contact with spirits. They were often the village elders. This was also a time when the medical profession was making its presence and power known in the new cities. They were also asserting their influence and power through the church. Do you know what the word 'witch' means? It means 'wise one'!"

"I didn't know that," I replied. "I actually have not read much on all of this."

"Well, if you're going to call yourself a religious historian, you might want to look into it!" Lee replied. "It's a long and sordid history of oppression and repression—and remember one more lesson from written history—it's written, for the most part, by the winners; the group in power, to justify themselves and their position.

"Anyway, most people lived in the country, and they were farmers and herdsmen. The city did not affect them and, as far as they were concerned, it was another world where they could occasionally go to sell their goods. They depended upon themselves and their villages for everything, including medicine and help of a spiritual nature. In each village, there was usually someone who had the power to diagnose and treat illness and solve personal problems. The people in the villages took care of these mostly elderly people because of their value to the community. The church's presence was there, but its hold was weak as people clung to their old ways. Many priests complained about their lack of power over these people, and the Inquisition was the result. These people were the village mystics, and, as such, were a threat to religious authority," Lee explained.

"What happened to them [mystics and healers]? Were they all killed?"

"Well, those that weren't, were driven underground or they learned to disguise their work as having other purposes. No, a lot were murdered or imprisoned, but many just went out of sight. Many were protected by their friends and family because they did help people. Did you know the word 'pagan' means 'a person from the country' and a 'heathen' means 'person of the heath'? They were the people not connected to the emerging cities and were thought of as politically unstable. The kings used the churches as a way of bringing these hillbillies, as we would say today, under some from of civil control. The medieval church also made the brilliant move of simply adopting the old pagan, sacred shrines, beliefs and even festivals, and giving them a Christian theme and focus. Old Saint Patrick was a master at this. He would simply declare a pagan shrine or well as Christian and assign a Christian saint to it. After that, the old village healer had to adapt his methods to the new religion just to survive.

"Let me read you something!" Lee added, fumbling through some papers. "Here it is. This is from a 1907 article in *Popular Science Monthly* entitled 'Magical Medical Practice in South Carolina' by John Hawkins:

> "'. . . as of that day, people of the German settlement of South Carolina still held to their traditional beliefs in healing and traced these beliefs to their pre-Christian origins. In old Germany neither Charlemagne's conquest nor the priest that followed it could put a period to the use of staves carved with mystic runes and devoted to the oak, the ash, and the willow preserved their sacred character; and in the old heathen formulas used for the cure of disease, the only change effected by Christianity was the substitution of the three highest names: (Father, Son and Holy Ghost) for those of Thor, Woden and other heathen deities.'"

"Pretty interesting, isn't it?" Lee said. "Anyway, the old beliefs adapted to their new authority and kept themselves secret. People developed a two-tiered system of religious authority despite continued efforts by the political and religious authorities to stamp out what they now termed as superstitious beliefs. That has continued to this day. People went to church and were good Christians, but they also went to the healer or hex when they needed to, and still do. As the church has cut itself off from the miraculous, and married its views with scientific rationalism, it has left a gap in the human life experience, that gap's where the mystic and healer still live."

"This is a lot to absorb," I remarked. "Could we take a break? Weren't we supposed to go somewhere?"

"Oh, yes, turn off your recorder and come with me."

We proceed out the front door and around the house to the woods. We walked quite a ways following a small stream that, due to recent rains, was babbling merrily. We reached a rock outcrop where Lee said, "Let's sit here for a while. I need to rest my feet."

We sat quietly, listening to the wind through the trees and watched as the sun flickered. It was a very peaceful, and my mind started to wander in a state of quietude. It felt as if the world was at peace.

"Do you feel it?" Lee softly asked, breaking in on my reverie.

"Feel what?" I whispered.

"The energies of this place" he replied, "This is a place of power. There is a presence here, a nature spirit. It's glad we're here."

"I do feel peaceful" I remarked, "but I'm not sure I feel anybody."

"Not a person." Lee sounded slightly annoyed. "A presence, a spirit. Come on, let's go." He stood up and starting walking on down the little trail.

I hurriedly got to my feet and toddled after him, feeling like I had failed to see the point and had disappointed him. As we walked along my mind settled back into the beauty of the morning and the quiet of the woods. I kept having the sense that something was following us, just out of sight and I found myself looking over my shoulder.

Lee noticed this and whispered, "You do feel it, don't you? You know he's following us, don't you?"

"Well, I feel something," I said. "Probably my imagination playing tricks on me."

"Is it indeed," he remarked." I supposed whatever it is would have to bite you in the ass before you'd believe it was there."

"I'm sorry," I apologized, "I'm just not used to seeing the world in this way. This is all pretty new to me."

"No harm done!" Lee replied. "I brought you out here to see if you could even sense a presence; and you can. It takes practice to be able to sense their presence and intent and to stop trying to rationalize everything you encounter. Let's head back to the house and have some lunch." He headed off in a determined fashion.

After we returned to his home and sat down to eat our sandwiches, I started the conversation again. "Okay, Lee, what was that in the woods?"

"I told you," he answered, "a presence, a spirit, a fairy, call it what you will!"

"A fairy?" I responded, "You mean like in fairy tales?"

"Not like children's fairy tales per se, but a presence, a consciousness that inhabits a place, a nature spirit. I'll bet you've sensed them before as a child, children don't have the mental blinders we adapt as we get older."

"Well, I suppose I did," I said, remembering all the little imaginary friends I had as an only child growing up and playing a great deal of the time alone. I had never seen my invisible playmates with my eyes I don't think, but I knew they were there. They had slowly faded away from my conscious mind as I got older, but I had never given it much thought. I suppose that many children's "invisible friends" could possibly be considered fairies, spirits or whatever. As I grew older, I learned that almost every child has had this kind of experience. Could it be that their minds and senses are more open to more subtle realms? Could it be that there was some actual, conscious presence? I used to hear them calling me by name as I played in my grandmother's backyard. Many times while hanging laundry, I thought I heard a mature female voice calling me. Knowing my grandmother meant business when she called me, I ran to the house only to find that she had not called me. This experience always left me puzzled and confused, until I started to recognize the difference between my grandmother's voice and my unseen friend. I remember trying to answer this friend, and, on one occasion, I was told I was hearing an angel, that she loved me but that I was to tell no one that she had spoken to me. After that, I would simply look up and smile in recognition. As a teenager and even into adulthood, I have heard that same female voice inside my head, loudly warning me of imminent dangers ranging from fights breaking out in bars, to dangerous people and situations, to being struck by cars running a red light and which I did not see. Who or whatever this entity is, it has saved my life on at least a dozen different occasions. I no longer worry about the who and the why, I just listen and obey.

"I guess its time we talked about spirits," Lee began. "Like this morning, in moments when sitting in the woods or by a lake or stream, did you find yourself turning around to find that no one was in your field of sight or caught a glimpse of something in your peripheral vision moving beside you? Did you ever hear faint voices or laughter in the silence of the deep woods and there was no other person around? Did you ever find yourself in a particular place becoming filled with an unknown terror and suddenly not recognizing the area with which you were formerly familiar? Well, you could simply pass all of this off as the product of an overactive imagination, or you could pay attention to these entities and learn a little something about the world of elementals or nature spirits."

Lee went on to explain that people in the past have referred to these spirits as fairies, gnomes, undines, elementals, dryads and a host of other names for the other less visible beings that also inhabit the natural world. He indicated that the early Spiritualists claimed that these entities have different levels of presence, awareness and tangibility.

Here is an interesting aside: About a year after this conversation with Lee, I received a call from an old high school friend that made me reflect on the potential power of these spirits of the natural world. This was an individual who, by anyone's account, was a practical, hard-working man, not given to flights of fancy, and in fact, was committed to the scientific explanation of the universe. This evening however, I could tell he was very agitated. The call went something like this:

"What's going on? Are you okay?" I asked.

"I need to talk to you. You know about these things!" he said. I had told him about some of my adventures with Lee.

"What things?"

"You know, like ghosts and that sort of thing," he replied.

"Okay, so what's got you all worked up?"

He continued, "Well, Cary, [his wife] dropped me off down at Tom's Creek to do some canoeing. I took my shovel and thought I'd look for some Indian artifacts to sell and make some money." (The Tom's Creek area is a swampy, snake-infested area just south of Columbia, South Carolina, where many Native American burial mounds exist. Sadly, many have fallen victim to "non-professional prospectors," like my friend.)

"I was down there in an area I'd been in before, when all of a sudden, I got completely disoriented. I thought I heard voices, and everything started to swirl. I got so shook up, I dropped my shovel and sack and ran to my canoe. I started paddling as fast as I could, but then I realized I was going in circles, and it was like something was after me. I started screaming and crying and begging to be left alone. My vision was blurred and I was totally panicked. Finally, I got my wits about me, my vision cleared and I paddled out of there to where Cary was to pick me up. What do you think happened?"

"Well, I can't say for sure, but it seems to me that something didn't want you out there digging in those burial mounds. You really should leave those places alone. It destroys all the evidence that the archeologists need to learn more about the Indians of that area. Are you going back to get your shovel?"

"Hell, no, they can have it!" he replied. "I'm never going back there again."

But to go back to my conversation with Lee. . . .

"You said in your book that spirits often find themselves, after death, wandering around in a state of confusion," I said.

"Oh, yes, because they are trained to expect themselves to be dead, and that's about the worst possible thing to happen to a person. For a long time, these spirits that I have here with me, two of them said that after they died, they thought they were supposed to be in their graves until Judgment Day, because that's what they'd been told in church. Then they got so restless and so dissatisfied that they thought they were supposed to be unconscious, too, and they weren't unconscious, and there's nothing worse than being in a grave and still conscious, I would imagine, even if you know your body's gone."

"So your actual personality is not unconscious," I ventured.

"It doesn't affect it in the least, but the beliefs do, and they [the spirits] thought, of course, that they were supposed to be unconscious, and they were for a while, and then it [the death experience] wore off. Just as soon as they came back to full awareness with six feet of dirt over them and hearing somebody up top, they wondered if Judgment Day was going on and they'd missed it," he said with a chuckle.

"Then they [the spirits] hear someone say up top, 'Well at least I got ten thousand dollars insurance out of it and that takes care of the funeral and gives me something to work on and I plan to get married next month anyway. . . .' So, just a little bit of that and they're not going to stay in their graves much longer, and here they come. Most people think that if they weren't in their graves they were supposed to be on the earth, just going back and forth all the time. The Boys [his spirits] talk about being on the road just like a bunch of hobos would, unless they can attach themselves to somebody, and then the next thing they want to do is to take up with somebody and become a familiar spirit. Like I say, I've got five of them, two here and three out in the yard."

"When you said that some of them needed a spirit to help them to a higher plane, what higher planes are you referring to?" I asked.

"Well, to a condition of being able to function as spirits, if nothing else, and accept the fact that they are dead. In many cases, they don't know that they are dead, just as in the case of Bridey Murphy. Bridey came back, wondering why her husband wouldn't pay any attention to her for a long time, and finally it dawned on her that she must be dead. This experience we call a universe is multilayered, and we are alive in many layers at once. Even our so-called past lives are still happening in one of those dimensions. Our individual consciousnesses are the one who create our higher and lower planes. A fellow spirit can and often does help us to see life at a higher plane . . . just like some people do here on this plane."

I noted to him that I had read a ghost story of a Confederate soldier who knew he was injured and went back home, and when he went into the kitchen where everybody was, no one would respond to him. Finally, he realized he was dead.

"I think that happens almost every time anytime dies in our system; they come back and wonder why people aren't paying them any attention anymore. Whenever I go past a grave that's just been made, and I think the person hasn't had a chance to be told of such things, I stop and I talk with the spirit that's there and tell them that it's all right, that they're dead, that they will get accustomed to the state they're in, and there's nothing to be afraid of, because they are just as much alive as they ever were. I tell them they will probably meet up with somebody soon [in spirit form] who will come along that will ease them across. . . . If they're lucky, they will. The terrible thing about that is, they see other spirits by their own light and with their own state of mind—their thoughts and beliefs. It's like I said in the book, about this spirit that we met the other night. The very same spirits that look to us like angels just scared other spirits out of their wits. That happens quite often," he said, "because this thing that was here the other night and was apparently in possession of Dick—one of the boys said it really was Lucifer, and I said 'Oh, I don't think so.' He said he thought it was Lucifer and that Dick thought it was and that gave him [the spirit] the shape it had. I can see that if the man concentrates and has a mental image of Lucifer and focuses that image on what's inside him, then whatever is inside him takes that shape, 'cause they follow the thought of the person that creates them, just as a piece of marble follows the chisel that cuts it out."

I thought about this for a bit. "Another thing occurs to me. In your book, the incident of the black nun, would that be referred to as a doppelganger?"

"I don't know what she is . . . I think she's an eidolon."

"An eidolon?" I wasn't familiar with this term.

Lee continued, "She was a manifestation of someone's anger, someone's hatred, resentment or guilt. I don't know what she was, but I do know they brought her into existence very soon after we came there, or activated her if she was already there and she was still there when I was young . . . I guess she's still there."

In an earlier conversation, Lee had talked about how an entity can take energy and tangibility from the presence of living people. It can, in a sense, recharge or empower itself, especially from strong emotions, like anger and fear, to the point of being detectable to those around it. Many times in, times of great emotional upheaval, a psychic part of ourselves can become disconnected from our physical being, and given the proper empowerment, will not dissipate but will take on a form of existence all its own.

"So you mean we create these eidolons?" I asked.

"Of course! We create our reality from our beliefs and emotions! The eidolon is just a bit that appears to be separated from us. One of the reasons we exist in a physical form is for our consciousness to learn to manage this ongoing creation of reality. Your whole life in this world is just a stage in the process!"

"Okay, what is a doppelganger, then?" I felt like we were getting off track.

"A doppelganger is a psychic double of the person that he can or some-times does involuntarily send out to do certain things. They said that my great-great-grandmother from West Virginia, Nancy, could send them out deliberately, and my Grandmother said she thought her grandfather could, also, to find out things for her. It's just going into a trance state, and letting a shape that looks like you, or would look like you if it met anybody, just go any place, find out and come back. I used to do it when I was boy just to find out things without having to go to the effort to go visiting. I was so fat, I hated to walk."

"I wish I could have done that," I said. "I was not only fat, but clumsy as a child."

"Oh, I was, too," he said, laughing. "I was falling down every time I turned around.

"You said you projected yourself as a child by holding your breath," I continued.

"I don't know exactly how I do it. I can hold my breath now, and I can't do it. The only time I do it now is accidentally. But there was just a little magic something, you'd hold your breath just right and look inward with your eyes, not focused on anything in particular, just looking in on yourself. . . . I don't know how to tell you, but you'd be moving on while your body was standing in a state of catalepsy."

Afterward I told Lee about a psychic experience I'd had as a teenager where, as I lay down on a couch to rest, I was, without warning, choked and repeatedly slapped by something I could touch but could not see. These incidents had only happened twice, but it had been years since then, without incident. I asked him if it was a poltergeist, thinking they must be associated with my adolescence because most poltergeist cases involve or occur in the presence of an adolescent. I had always wondered what that was, because the two incidents occurred within a few weeks of each other, and I still don't sleep on the couch. On both occasions, I was tired, but relaxed and in a good mood. Lee asked me if I'd been upset, and I said no.

"Then I don't think it would be a poltergeist," he said. "They don't usu-ally behave like that. That sounds like a low-grade spirit of some kind that really has a consciousness. Poltergeists, I don't think, have a consciousness."

Parallel Worlds

Lee taught me that human beings, once their physical life has ended, merely cross over (a term often used by Spiritualists to describe the process of death) and assume a less tangible form of themselves in a parallel dimension. He explained that all life is conscious energy, embodied or not, existing in various phases of physical density from solid, like a human being, to the very subtle forms of tangible thought forms. Little children can often detect their presence before they are taught to ignore such occurrences, or they'll appear odd to the modern world and cause their parents embarrassment.

"Can you imagine? If some child starts talking about talking fairies or little people at dinner in front of the whole family? Why, the parents would be reprimanded for allowing such behavior, and the child would be suspect from that moment onward, branded a kook, a weirdo or worse. Why, they'd lock him up!"

I had to admit, he was correct, that society as a whole did not accept this once common behavior. Sadly, I reflected that this was not a time for the visions and revelations on which most of our religious traditions and history are based. It just would not be accepted or allowed.

Lee continued, "If you practice being still in your body and in your mind, and allowing yourself to recognize what your inner mind is sensing, your mind will gradually begin to open its awareness of these subtle forms of energy that surround us all the time. It also means opening your awareness to the fields of energy that flow in and through this earth as the dynamic forces of nature. Gradually, you become aware of these entities in the natural world and how they not only can, but do, interact with you, for better or for worse."

"But why is it so hard to physically see them?" I asked.

"You can see them if you relearn how! You'll just have to unlearn what you've been taught and open yourself up to their presence."

"Yeah," I replied, "but, how come some people can easily see them and most can't?"

"Their senses are just more attuned" Lee said. "Look at the dog or cat. They can hear frequencies that we can't. Have you ever seen one of those special silent whistles? You blow it and you'd think nothing was happening and then Rover starts barking. His ears are just more attuned and some gifted people are more attuned to the presence of spirits. That doesn't mean with practice, you can't detect them also.

"This world we live and exist in is like the layers of an onion, multi-layered and multidimensional. There are worlds even beyond the one they [spirits] inhabit, in almost endless layers of reality. Most of the entities we call ghosts are merely entities from this dimension that exist in immediate proximity to our own. They exhibit all the characteristics of those that inhabit this one."

"Are they more spiritually advanced than we are?" I asked.

Lee laughed and said, "You assume that because they are not bound by gross bodies that they are not subject to the same feelings and emotions and foibles of the physical mind. They have consciousness, will and desires, hates and joys as we do."

Lee often cautioned that many people who assume that these entities speak for higher powers have brought themselves and their friends much embarrassment by prattling on about the greater nature of things eternal. Spirits, he would say, will feed you a line of bull as quickly as the next person. Use your common sense when dealing with spirits; if they say something that sounds like crap, it probably is.

Lee continued, "The majority of spirits you meet in forests, at streams or other natural places are childlike, harmless and in fact, playful, as long as they and their environs are given proper respect. They will often follow you through the woods at a short distance, and you often notice their rustling in dry leaves, or you become aware of their presence as a quick movement out of the corner of your eye. Every once in a while one will attach itself to you and follow you home."

Lee sat back into his rocker and lit his pipe. "Let me tell you a story of a famous nature spirit from around here. We used to call him Old Bunkum, and he was a nature spirit that followed and annoyed a local elderly farmer during his life and even after his death. One of Old Bunkum's most famous pranks was to muss the hair of the old man, who prided himself in his neat appearance. Many friends and family of the old man watched in amazement as the old man's hair would become disarrayed before their eyes, usually at dinner. The poor old fellow would curse, excuse himself and go comb his hair in the bathroom. Toward the end of his life, the pranks took an even more bizarre twist, as exemplified by one traumatic incident that occurred during a hunting trip. It seems that the old farmer had gone hunting, and needing to answer the call of nature, stopped in the field and proceeded to relieve himself. It was at this point that Old Bunkum appeared and grabbed the old man's private parts. Terrified, the old man screamed, dropped his rifle and to the amazement of those with him, began running and screaming across the field in the direction of his home. Upon reaching home, he locked himself in his room and hid in his bed under the covers. The shock was too much for him, and he died in a matter of days. At his funeral, the mourners observed a ball of light enter the living room via a window where the casket was being displayed, saw it bounce along the casket and muss the hair of the recently deceased, one last time. Aside from sending the mourners into hysterics, this was the last time anyone witnessed the pranks of Old Bunkum."

"That is quite a story," I responded. "So not all nature spirits are peaceful and friendly?"

"No indeed," Lee said. "That's a belief from the turn of the last century when they had a wave of interest in fairies in Victorian England. You know, fairies were not tiny and winged until Shakespeare made them so in *A Mid-Summer Night's Dream*. You should read that sometime, you'll find it fascinating."

Lee's mention of Victorian England reminded me of a particular circumstance where these non-human entities could be summoned to human presence with rituals and incantations, such as this chant from Sussex for summoning fairies. Holding a specially prepared wand, the person who wished to summon and encounter fairies, would, at dusk, chant:

> Come in the stillness, come in the night,
> Come soon and bring delight.
> Beckoning, beckoning left hand and right,
> Come now, Come now, come tonight.

Many of these cunning folk of Ireland, Scotland, Wales, and England relied heavily upon their ability to effectively communicate with these spirits to perform their cures, make their charms and conduct their magical affairs. As a result, they were known as fairy doctors.

There are numerous tales of the fairy doctors/cunning folk. Many asserted that their knowledge of the supernatural and of their healing ability came from the realm of fairy, a world coexisting with ours and yet invisible to our normal vision. Cunning men spoke of their journeys to this dimension of spirits, and the knowledge from that world they brought back to the physical world.

This shamanic ability to travel between these worlds and return with information and knowledge from the spirit world was a highly valued individual in the past. One of the most famous of these people was a 19th-century Irish cunning woman from east County Clare, known widely as Biddy Early. Mistress Early claimed that many of her powers were learned from listening at a fairy fort. She claimed to have been gifted with a special spirit bottle that allowed her to diagnose illness and to see things at a distance. Although in direct defiance of the local priests and bishop, Biddy Early was a highly respected and much-sought-after healer until her death in 1873. In his book *The Middle Kingdom: The Faerie World of Ireland*, Diarmuid MacManus says that in true shamanic tradition, Biddy Early accepted no payment for her healing and thus never rose from her life of comparative poverty (Mac Manus, 1993, 158). Throughout her life, she was known to consult with the spirit world on her healings, had visionary experiences and knew how to interpret and evaluate their communications.

Studying this subject, as I have now for many years, I have found that people often do not realize that in most cultures of the world there exist tales of such entities and their activities in the world of humans. The Native Americans of the Cherokee tribe had tales of a mostly invisible race of small people, or Yundi Tsundi, who lived in certain sections of the forest or caves and who were afforded great deference and respect to avoid misfortune. Throughout much of human history, these entities were of human size and even appeared as giants when needed.

Most spirits, Lee would say, have no need to make themselves known to us, as most of us cannot respond to their presence. Spirits can and do, on occasion, enter the world of dreams and visions when the human mind is attuned to them. The most appropriate state of mind for sensing them is one of quiet alertness. You can practice getting into this state by meditation, dance, walking, and even singing.

According to Lee, you learn and practice opening yourself to the spirit world through ritual, meditation or other vehicles. Once contact is made, proceed with caution, common sense, and always with respect for what you find. I have always found their presence a somewhat comforting reminder that physical death is only the beginning of our long journey homeward. Lee would often say that dealing with Elementals/spirits is not without danger; yet, if you can manage it, it can provide you with amazing experiences and teach you many things.

Here is what Lee meant by opening yourself to other worlds or dimensions of reality. Being a shaman means being able to, at will, alter one's consciousness and open new fields and avenues of perception. The major way for a shaman or Powwow practitioner to heal or to operate in the world of spirit is to enter various levels of trance. In light trance, the channel from the Divine will open and the healing will take place while the Powwow is still in a relatively normal state of awareness. In deeper trance, however, the Powwow easily loses the awareness of the world, and several levels of perception may present themselves. These added levels of perception are difficult to describe, but often include:

1. **The ability to be fully absorbed in your inner awareness of and within the present moment.** At this level of awareness, the past and future are not apart of your consciousness as they are normally as we mentally bounce back and forth all the time in our daily activities between the considerations of each for perspective. In this state, we are more aware of what's around us, to the point that the regular world becomes slightly unreal, like a dreamscape. People and things seem to be moving as figures in a motion picture. They often appear hollow, as you realize that you, too, are part of an infinite, ongoing process. Your normal, everyday personality, with all its needs, motivations, agendas, etc., is like everything else: a bundle of constructs that are often mistaken for reality by your awareness. The personal experience of this highly focused state of awareness can have a profound effect on your life. You cannot and should not try to pursue your

daily activities while in this mental state, it is simply not practical for everyday activities. You must practice and learn to switch back and forth between these different states of awareness to do your shamanic work and still remain a viable member of society. To be able to reach this sort of awareness, however, is very useful for performing healings in the Powwow tradition and is critical for spirit-related activities and interactions. Some shamans employ prayer, meditation, chanting, drumming and dancing to achieve a similar heightened state of awareness.

2. **The interdependency of all things.** Another characteristic that occurs in a deep trance state is the interdependency of all things, each interacting and affecting the other. The metaphor of the world inside the aquarium is appropriate and approximates this state of trance. In such a mental state, you realize quickly that your thoughts, and even the slightest movement, can impact and effect change far beyond the normally accepted sphere of a human. Also, you can move the energy you generate through this interconnected aquarium universe. It is within this flow that magical acts and spirit contacts are possible.

3. **Everyday events are seen as one sum and substance.** Everyday events and occurrences, while appearing different, are now seen as explicitly one sum and substance. Whatever you do in this environment will eventually affect you and those around you; therefore, acts of hatred and violence, even psychic violence, will eventually find their way back to you. This understanding affects the actions of a shaman. You realize that everyone is always in a process of becoming; that the future is, at best, an idea. This experience can be for some people psychologically comforting and for others emotionally disturbing. One disturbing impact of this realization for many novice shamans is that you realize that you are constantly creating your inner reality. You are creating your fate with your thoughts, internal dialogues and even with your subtle mental states. As other entities are also a part of this process, their thoughts are also impacting the total process and affecting you as well. Your personal, subtle system of cause and effect can actually be internally felt, and you become aware of the moments

at which you are altering your course for better or worse. This, too, can be an unsettling experience at first but can, over time, serve as an internal alert system to those who choose to listen for it. In deep trance states, you also become aware of an internal and eternal flow of energy within yourself and in all things. Most often, it is experienced by your conscious mind as a form of light, or it can be physically felt as a form of liquid moving in and through all things.

You may be saying to yourself, well, so what? Isn't this known already from mystical writings in the past? The answer is, of course, yes. The problem with just reading about something is the lack of personal interaction and experience. If everything just lives at the cognitive, analytical level of the brain, it may be understood, but it will not have the same impact on you as a person. I once knew an individual who, due to life circumstances, had never personally seen the ocean. When she finally did, the impact of the experience she described was so profound it brought tears to her eyes as she described the waves and their movement.

Struggling with Acceptance

This was not the end of my discussions or encounters to the world of spirits. Lee Gandee lived most of his days during that period of his life immersed in a world of the unseen as well as the visual. Like shamans of old, he treated both as we treat the visual world. Now, you may be asking yourself, was this man crazy, delusional or just taking this kid on a mind trip? How can anyone, in this day and age, possibly believe in such things? Believe me, I asked myself these and many other questions repeatedly throughout the experiences I had. I wondered about Lee Gandee, Sheriff McTeer and Mrs. Ramsey, the Granny-woman. I also wondered how what I had experienced would be perceived by my professors and peers as I wrote my thesis. Nothing in my formal anthropological, religious, or folk studies had prepared me for such an unexpected and strange level of involvement in these shamanic traditions.

In "The Reality of Spirits," published in 1997 in *Shamanism*, respected anthropologist Edith Turner tackled the issue of Western intellectual imperialism historically inherent in the discipline: "In the past in anthropology, if a researcher "went native," it doomed him academically" (1). She observed that this distance was common among many field researchers. "This is how we thought. Little knowing it, we denied the people's equality with ours, their 'coevalness,' their common humanity as that humanity extended itself into the spirit world" (1).

As she became more involved with various native peoples, Turner began to doubt the authenticity of the usual anthropological fieldworker's stance:

> And I began to see how anthropologists have perpetuated an endless series of put-downs about the many spirit events in which they participated—"participated" in a kindly pretense. They might have obtained valuable material, but they have been operating with the wrong paradigm, that of the positivists' denial. (1)

Turner goes on to chide the discipline's past by noting,

> Members of many different societies, even our own, tell us they have had experience of seeing or hearing spirits. Let us recall how anthropology has dealt with the question in the past. (3)

> Mainline anthropologists have studiedly ignored the central matter of this kind of information—central in the people's own view—and only used the material as if it were metaphor or symbol, not reality, commenting that such and such "metaphor" is congruent with the function, structure, or psychological mind set of the society. Clearly, this is a laudable endeavor as far as it goes. But the neglect of the central material savors of our old bête noire, intellectual imperialism. (3)

Turner also ponders how students of anthropology should view the variety of spirit worlds from different cultures:

> "Is this kind of subject matter logical anyway? Have we the right to force it into logical frameworks? I would assert that if we are to understand the fullness of the experiences that occurred during these interviews, it is impossible and somewhat disingenuous to subject the experiences to the reality grid of the modern scientific mind. It simply doesn't fit the framework and too much information is lost in the process." (4).

Once after a lecture to a college class, I was asked if I thought that "all of this stuff on nature spirits and spirits in general could just be explained as aspects of human consciousness, and imagination?" I replied that I did, but on the other hand, I asked the class if anyone in the room could give me an exhaustive and comprehensive definition of human consciousness and imagination? The room fell silent. To paraphrase the philosopher Schopenhauer, each person takes the limits of his or her intellectual and physical vision to constitute the totality of the world. So each of us has the tendency to view the world through our own sensory, cultural and intellectual limits and distrusts that which appears outside those limits. It's a safe and secure posture, and for most of us, serves as a lifelong assurance that the things of this world exist just as we have been informed.

I cannot but reflect on the history of medical innovation, and in particular, the discovery of the presence of germs, viruses, and the microscopic world in general. Those persons who initially asserted that infection and disease could have, as its causes, physical forms that could not be seen with the naked eye or the current technology of the era, were openly ridiculed. In some cases, the proponents of such ideas were driven from their very professions by the academic establishment of the day. As soon as devices were designed to reveal this inner world, opinion began to change slowly. It seems, in light of past history, that while no one should accept, unquestioningly, the presence of a parallel universe or the presence of disembodied entities in our field of consciousness, we should endeavor to keep an open mind to the possibility that we simply may not yet have a tool to objectively verify their existence. To simply dismiss outright the possibility of such possibilities, based on the lack of physical evidence, is, in a sense, arrogant, ignorant and also ignores the record of history. Such thinking reveals a fear of the existence of things that we may not be able to control.

The issue of an alternate reality gave me endless consternation during the fieldwork and afterward. I finally had to make a choice to just experience and describe, suspending analysis and judgment until some later date when I had better tools with which to view the evidence. As you will see later in this book, events occurred that challenged and altered my limited view of the world. As a result, I simply turned the experience into a paper on the history of these shamanic traditions and let it go at that. To an extent, I am still suspending final judgment with much of the esoteric elements and events. I am leaving it up to each of you to interpret these people and experiences as you see fit. Just keep in mind the lessons of history before pronouncing your final sentence.

Getting Used to Lee's Abilities and the Presence of Spirits

These encounters with a world unseen continued throughout the span of the study and my relationship with Lee Gandee. The world of spirit was, as I stated earlier, one that he took very seriously. In another interview, we were discussing local people who practiced Hexerei when, from the corner of my eye, I caught sight of something in the south-facing window in Lee's room. As my attention was diverted, I witnessed a luminous ball, the size of a mature grapefruit, enter the room, float along the mantelpiece and float out the window on the other side of the room.

Needless to say, I was awestruck, until I heard Lee say, "Jack, are you listening to me?" I turned to face him, and he added, "You saw that, didn't you?"

I nodded and exclaimed, "What was that?"

"Nothing really, just one of my boys coming in to see what was going on. You'll have to get used to seeing things like that if you're going to be coming around here."

I had an unsettled and anxious feeling as I tried to move on with the interview and kept peeking at the window. I have since realized that when some event occurs that appears outside the realm of ordinary reality, this feeling of disorientation and anxiety is commonplace. It results from our mind's attempts to process something it was not expecting to encounter. I did witness similar luminous balls appear and move around in Lee's house after that day. These luminous balls moved, sometimes with apparent intelligent purpose, and I always found them a bit unnerving, although I learned to tolerate their presence. St. Elmo's fire? My hallucination? Static electricity? Disembodied entities? I didn't have a clue. In those early days, it is important to note that I initially observed these phenomena only while in Lee's house or property, and this led me to think that there was some unique connection between Gandee and these manifestations. I soon learned that suspicion was *not* borne out by experience. Lee's home was probably just a more open environment for these phenomena.

Lee explained the presence of spirit entities metaphysically by saying that all matter was simply a condensation of energy; that energy could be neither created nor destroyed, only endlessly reconstituted and reformed, which was at least a familiar concept from early science classes. The universe and everything in it, as we know and experience it, Lee believed, is composed of condensed matter formed by the energy of Divine thought. We are, as humans, simply more physically dense versions of this Divine energy than are those entities in the spirit world. They are, so to speak, less tangible than we are, and yet, still embody awareness of some sort.

Thoughts can and do take on a life of their own as ideational constructs in ever-increasing degrees of density. This is, as I've said before, the principle behind magical healing. To be able to envision and focus one's mental energy on something is to effect some change, even at a subtle level. Thought, in this scheme, shares a similar metaphysical role as the Hindu conception of Shakti or primal energy. In this view, Shakti gives matter its dynamic quality, without which it would be simply inert. In the final sense, we are all manifestations of a universal conscious mind, existing within that consciousness.

As discussed earlier, shamans have always had the cultural role of intermediary and communicator to the world of spirit. The root doctor performed his communication with the spirit world while in a trancelike state. In some cases, his diagnosis of the person's illness was made by entering the patient's body in spirit form. This method parallels activities employed by shamanic practitioners in many cultures, where spirits are drawn to the shaman's enhanced awareness, and after attaching themselves to the practitioner, the spirits then became the shaman's daily companions and assistants. Gandee called these spirits his "boys."

Gandee's boys were not just spirit companions but were also essential to his work as a Hexenmeister. In his youth, Gandee said that he developed and practiced projecting his consciousness out of his body to go wandering. In his autobiography, *Strange Experience: Secrets of a Hexenmeister*, Lee chronicles these activities and his grandmother's disapproval, on the grounds that a malevolent spirit might seize the opportunity and occupy his body. Once occupied, the spirit could, acting as Gandee, commit mischief, for which Gandee would have to suffer. The concept of possible intrusion or possession of a shaman while in a trance state by a hostile spirit is a common belief among shamanic practitioners worldwide.

Gandee's spirits or boys, therefore, had clearly defined roles. Their most commons roles were that of investigator and reporter of activities at a distance. When he needed to know some information not readily available, instead of sending his own consciousness, he sent one of the spirits, who would make the journey and then report back on what had been seen. Most often, a client would ask for some information on a missing relative, traveling spouse, or distant friend. Gandee would send one of his boys (spirits) to investigate and then relay to the client at a later date what had been reported to him.

"I'm just getting too old to go myself and it's a lot easier to send one of the boys," he once remarked to me. In this manner, he also protected himself against unwelcome spirit intrusions from which he had suffered both physically and emotionally in the past. Gandee, when preparing to enter trance, would secure the assistance of a knowledgeable and trusted companion to watch over and protect his physical form while his consciousness went elsewhere in search of specific information or individuals. He would lie upon his bed and enter trance. His body would stiffen to the point of rigidity; his breathing would become shallow. The person watching over him was to watch for irregularities in his trance state and was prepared to protect him, should a non-resident spirit attempt to enter his body. In the times that I performed this service for him, I never observed such an event. Still, upon returning to his body and normal state of awareness, he would be exhausted and often need to be helped to his feet and given liquids before he could speak of his venture. More commonly, he would send one of his boys' spirits to seek the information and then communicate with them upon their return. This phenomenon was called "knowing at a distance."

The incidence of knowing at a distance was brought home to me in a very disconcerting manner during one of our earliest interviews.

"One of my boys was over at your place last night. He says your girlfriend is quite pretty," Lee said to me casually.

"Oh," I responded, "and what did he say she looks like?" I knew Gandee had never seen the girl I was then dating.

"Well, he says she's petite, with brown hair and hazel eyes and a cute figure, though her breasts are smaller than he likes. He says you two were getting frisky last night."

I blushed at the forward nature of his comment and attempted to counter with, "Oh, well, if he thinks he saw something, then tell me what he said happened," knowing the only window to our bedroom was some thirty feet from the ground. To my shock and humiliation, Lee went on to describe in detail the sequence of events of the previous night as if he had been standing in the room.

I sat in stunned silence as he said, "You still think all of this is just some sort of game, don't you? Something you can treat with your scholarly detachment and it won't affect you, but magic is real, and the deeper you go, the more ready you'd better be for what happens. If you can't take the heat, get out of the kitchen!"

"I understand," I responded meekly. "I do take this seriously; it's just I have to go back to the world where these things don't happen."

"Oh, but they do happen," he quickly responded. "You're just not aware of it."

On the way home that day, I resolved never to mention to my girl-friend what had transpired, as I knew she would be as unnerved as I was and paranoid about our privacy in the future. I know I was self-conscious for a long time afterward.

To return to the transcript of our taped interviews, here is where we left off: "So all spirits are not necessarily ghosts of people who once lived?" I asked.

"No, indeed," Lee replied. "There are as many types of spirits as there are types of awareness. Even places, buildings and things can develop a form of consciousness; many plants and trees have a form of awareness, not to mention animals. So why wouldn't the spirit world be the same? Have you ever noticed the energy in the sanctuary of a church?"

"Yes, but I could not make sense out of it; it seemed jumbled and confused."

Lee agreed. "Exactly. Look at all the different feelings and emotions that are expressed and then left there: guilt, anger, joy sorrow; all of which leave a residue in the building that a sensitive person can detect."

Lee's comment reminded me of an interesting anecdote, so I recounted the story of a friend who, while touring a castle in England, had become separated from the tour and found himself in a room he did not recognize, but which inexplicably filled him with panic and terror. When he raced from the room and rejoined the tour, he asked the guide about the room and was told it was where prisoners were tortured.

At this point, Lee interrupted me. "This emotional energy, conscious or otherwise, remains present like a dust that is picked up by others who encounter it. This residue has much to do with the phenomena of ghosts. Spirits who once had human form often are not aware of their change of circumstances. . . . They don't realize they are dead! This is why it is the duty of the Powwow to go and sit by a fresh grave and talk to the spirit."

"What would you say?" I asked him.

"Well, I would first let him know that I know he's dead and that he needs to realize that he's dead," Lee replied. "Some of them try to lie there in the casket and wait for the Rapture. Just tell them not to be afraid, to come on out of the coffin and that if they wait, some spirit will be along to help them with their new life. I tell them that this new life will be unlike their old one and that they will need some help adjusting. Sometimes they even go back to their former home, only to discover that their families can't hear or see them. Sometimes, they find out what their families really thought of them and how much they really cared. That's a revelation for them! I tell them not to be upset if those of us still in human form can't see them to respond to them."

"Why can't I see these spirits?" I asked.

"Because they are vibrating at a level that is too fast for us to see with the naked eye. At best, we might catch a glimpse of them out of the corner of our eye unless we are a trained medium, like the spiritualists. They are specially trained to open that part of their mind to be able to see spirits," Lee said.

"Can you personally see them? Can you hear them?"

"Of course," Lee replied, lighting his pipe. "As clearly as I see and hear you now, in that chair . . . and I can feel their touch as well."

"That would give me the creeps!" I looked around nervously. "Pretty soon you would not know what was real and what was not!"

Lee replied in a serious but bemused tone. "It's all real, but you learn to know the difference and how to screen them out when you don't want to interact. Right now, one of my boys is standing behind you, but he knows not to show himself, as it would probably send you over the edge if he did. You're just not ready."

I looked quickly over my shoulder and, of course, saw nothing. "Okay, Lee, but what does all of this mean?" I tried to regain my composure. "What does this world of spirits and entities mean in terms of God and spirituality? How does it benefit you in an ultimate sense, in terms of your soul?"

He chuckled. "You amaze me with your questions. Sometimes I can see you've got it and then sometimes you retreat back to your ordinary mindset and come up with some question that shows you're still refusing to see what's right in front of you.

"What does it mean in terms of God and spirit?" Lee continued. "It means your little world, your little reality is so much wider and deeper than you can imagine; it's so much more than this ordinary world, so much deeper than you have been led to believe. It means we live in multiple realities endlessly and at the same time. It means that God is not separate from you and your so-called soul, and in the end, God is the only thing that is real. Life itself is God's experience; you and I and the spirits are just ideas, just part of his endless dreaming. Life is the result of God's desire to live, to experience, to interact. It means you are so much more than this life, this physical self, and your mind is always changing, always in the process of becoming. It means that all this is so much more than concepts like good and evil, heaven and hell, like in religions. Religions are mankind's attempt to put controls and restraints on the human experience of God. . . . So they organize and codify and finally manage to tell you that only they have the truth, and if you're a good boy and listen to everything they say, that you'll be rewarded for your obedience with some paradise in the sky. In the end, you spend your life in church committees, planning socials, begging for forgiveness and doing everything you can to keep from really experiencing the reality of God. In the end, when your spirit wakes in the grave, it's

confused and disoriented. Some other spirit has to come along and help it
with its new realm of existence."

I was fascinated by this new perspective and tried to absorb these ideas.
I must have looked a bit puzzled, because Lee then said, "Jack, you should
know by now that this existence or life you are currently experiencing does
not end in so-called death," Lee continued. "It only changes form. Your life
is contained in your consciousness of it. Remember when we were talking
about being aware that you are dreaming while you are dreaming? Remember how you have learned to observe your own dreams? Who is observing
that dream? Jack Montgomery? Lee Gandee? No, something far deeper
and more wonderful, something timeless, wonderfully alive, wonderfully
aware. . . . You can't die because your real self never stopped existing.

"In the next world," Lee continued, "the spirit world, you are not bound
by the same physical form, but that same you that watches your dreams is
looking through its new vehicles of perception. You learn and experience a
different type of existence, one where physical form and distance mean nothing. We are the embodiment of God's longing to experience self-awareness
and evolve. All creation is an expression of this evolution. Even in the spirit
world, away from the grossness of a material existence, that growth is still
taking place all the time. "All of this," he added softly, meaning Powwow, "is
a method, a way to experience all these things in this time and space; while
you are in this form, you can realize that you are so much more than you
ever thought. That your mind and awareness can, instead of limiting you,
set you free; it can open your eyes and mind to what is really there. Does
that make any sense to you?"

"I think so," I replied. "I need to think about it for a while."

"You do that," he replied. "I know you have the potential to see, if you
let yourself."

In the end, he was right, of course, but it would be years before I realized the full meaning of his words.

Additional Thoughts on These Experiences

In Lee's view, his particular spirits do not automatically re-enter human
forms. Many continue to evolve toward more subtle forms of existence, in
other more abstract dimensions, where thought and state of awareness are

everything. All the while they're moving back toward the ultimate awareness we call the Divine or God—without form or name. By this time, they are way beyond our ability to perceive them while in an embodied state. The ones we can most commonly encounter are, in a sense, our neighbors next door, just one step beyond our own. Spirits elect sometimes to return to an embodied form. This is the process called reincarnation, where spirits return to a physical body through rebirth to finish that which was unfinished in their previous life or for whatever need draws them back. This is why, for myself, after years of encountering these entities, it no longer has the appeal or novelty it once had when I first began this study.

Lee once told me that spirits are also, like their embodied counterparts, composite in nature. You are not just one person; you're the sum of endless incarnations, endless lives. You get some of it from your parents and some of it from those endless lives.

Science has yet to confirm the existence or acknowledge this form of biological memory. Thomas McClaskey, writing for the American Academy of Experts in Traumatic Stress in "Decoding Traumatic Memory Patterns at the Cellular Level," says, "Virtually every behavioral pattern exhibited during routine activities of daily living results from learned data which is stored, or encoded, as cellular memory" (1). McClaskey adds that "In a condition such as Post Traumatic Stress Disorder, it must be kept in mind that the 'problem' is an expression of traumatically encoded information at the cellular level" (1).

Spirits, Lee said, tell us that this body we have now is only the box in which we make our appearance in the physical world. It's not meant to last but its contents are. The physical body is a product of the physical world; you get it from your parents and all those who came before. You spirit comes to it from the other dimension, carrying all the dust of lessons learned and not learned from previous lives, and re-enters the physical world. Your physical body lives because your spirit comes into it, and what you are is a product of that union. That combination is your heritage, and it becomes your thoughts, tendencies, likes, dislikes and so on. Then, after you live this life, your spirit leaves this world again with all the lessons gained from it, until it decides to take another birth, stay where it is or evolve onto a higher realm.

The Second Sight

The ability to detect the presence of a more subtle entity takes considerable practice for most of us, and once mastered, needs to be managed to avoid becoming a distracting nuisance. After years of being able to detect their presence, and on occasion engage in communication, much of the initial fascination has waned, and I find myself just speaking as if passing some-one on the street and going about my regular business. On occasion, as I mentioned earlier an entity has intruded to alert me to danger in my life. Most recently, while going to the grocery store, I was about to pull away from an intersection when I heard a female voice exclaim, "Jack, stop the car!" I instantly hit the brakes in time to see a truck whiz by, through the red light, without stopping. I caught my breath and whispered, "Thanks, I really appreciate it!" I have been saved from many other dangerous events and people in this manner. It has happened so many times that when I hear them speak, I listen and appreciate their kind acts.

In terms of Powwow, it is believed that you get many of your abilities, tendencies, subtle memories and preference from the merging of physical and spirit-based memories that further suggests the origin of your composite nature from life to life. Either way, your personality or the details of your life do not result from some Divine administrative judgment, but as the result of a complex natural process.

If you are resolute in learning to enhance your awareness so you can sense and communicate with these more subtle forms of existence, you need to do the following:

You must patiently practice opening yourself in small increments to the presence of more subtle forms of energy by meditating, entering trance, prayer or other means. All of the methods work in time and with diligence. You are learning to "read" energy.

First, become familiar with your own energy field by holding your palms facing each other and learning to detect the energy flowing between them and through your body. As time and your practice progresses, you will start to be able to detect the energy of others. To do this, find someone you know and practice sensing his or her energy. Pretty soon, you will be able to have them pass you without being in your field of vision and know they are present as they enter the house or room.

You'll discover that each person's energy is like a fingerprint, a signature. Usually, people learning to do this sort of sensing will go out in public with their psychic energy still extended and become overwhelmed by the intensity and variety of energies. To be effective and maintain your mental equipoise, you must practice shutting off this enhanced state of awareness. I have always loved antiques and going to antique stores and malls, but after several learning experiences, I now avoid touching or handling things carelessly in stores, and especially in antique shops. While new merchandise usually has no residue of energy on it, antiques are often saturated with human energy residues.

In short, when you are out in public, you must not open yourself fully. You can, so to speak, keep a small light on for protection. I was at a party, relaxing, and unconsciously opened myself. As I was introduced to a rather plain-looking individual whose hand I shook, I was seized with an awareness that is was not someone with whom I wanted to associate. He seemed to sense my awareness and stared intently at me. I politely and quickly found a way to exit the conversation, shielded myself psychically and moved to another room. Later, I learned that this individual had been convicted of child molestation. To put it bluntly, his energy was evil. Now, most of the time, even out in public, I keep a certain kind of awareness open, for self-protection. It proves very useful and has never steered me wrong.

Another excellent way to experience enhanced awareness is to spend time in complete solitude, preferably in silence. Nature is a wonderful setting for such an experience. Walking in deep woods, sitting alone by the seashore or canoeing by yourself down a quiet stream or river are ideal. Rent a cabin in the woods, leave all your electronic noisemakers and distracters at home or turn them off and store them out of sight. Get used to the silence, hearing only your thoughts and breath. Don't sing or talk, just sit and listen. Gradually you will begin to hear and sense in a way you had forgotten or never knew existed. As you delve deeper into the silence, your talking mind will shut down its incessant rambling, and you will awaken to an awareness you can barely imagine. Revel in it; there is much wisdom in that silence. Move through the woods as silently as possible, and your consciousness will start to expand outwardly. At this time, trust the impressions you receive. All this will get you used to the states of heightened awareness necessary for spirit contact in a safe and controlled manner. One friend who has led a very urban, harried life told me he found himself sobbing at the beauty he found in his solitude. He felt the presence of something he took to be an angel enveloped him in its arms, and he felt like a baby once again. All of this may sound very simple, but most of real spirituality is like that. No need for complex rituals or chanted verses; you are only encountering what has always been there.

It is important to take this process of raising your awareness as a very serious matter. Above all, do not use mind-altering substances of any kind. If you are currently undergoing psychiatric treatment or have a condition for which you must take medication to stabilize your emotions and thoughts, do not engage in this process. While a substance may open a door to enhanced perception quickly, you may not be ready for what appears to you or be able to close the door if needed. Shamanic journeying and enhanced perception are psychological arts, and require practice to develop the skills needed to enact them successfully. Using some substance to accelerate your growth is playing with fire, and you will get burned.

If you are physically ill and hoping to help heal yourself, this is not a time to practice your shamanic skills. You will need all your strength and awareness to be able to practice successfully and safely. I have known those who tried to do this practice under the influence of drugs. The results were uniformly disastrous, even if they appeared to succeed initially. I know that some will say, "Oh, I read that shamans in such-and-such a culture use substances like peyote to induce visions, and they seem to come to no harm!" To these folks, I say, "Correct, but you were not raised in such a culture and you are not from a culture that is conducive and accepting of this method of vision-seeking. Look around you at those from our culture who engage in long-term use of these substances. Do you want to end up like that?" There is just no need in this culture to walk that particular path of drug use as a shaman. You can do it on your own, without using any substances. The results will be more rewarding without drugs, and your physical and mental health won't be compromised.

Once you can open yourself to more subtle forms of energy, you will need to be able to discern actual encounters from your personal fantasies and daydreams. This skill will help to keep you safe and from going off on psychological tangents. It is very difficult to describe how a real encounter differs, but once you have experienced it, you will know. The simplest analogy is that your fantasies are like casual dreaming that flits from episode to episode and has little impact on you. An encounter, while often in trance, is more profoundly real and can even manifest physically.

For example, when I first moved to Virginia, I was often teased and annoyed by what seemed to be a playful imp as I would try to rest. It would scamper onto the bed, pull at my sheets and otherwise torment me. At first, I believed it to be a hypnagogic hallucination, as it occurred when I was trying to fall asleep. Finally, one day, in frustration, I grabbed at it and caught it in my hand. It was like grabbing an invisible monkey's arm. All of a sudden, it bit me and a sharp stinging pain soared up my arm and brought me to a full waking state. As I looked down at my hand, I noticed that I had a horseshoe-shaped bite that was red and inflamed. I rushed to the bathroom and applied antiseptic. I then tore apart my small apartment bedroom to make certain I was physically alone. I bandaged my hand and set about psychically cleansing the room, which is what I should have done in the first place. The incident never repeated itself, and my hand suffered no permanent harm.

As an epilogue, I accidentally ran into a fellow graduate student in a local bar who had rented the same room, several years before I had. I asked him how he liked the apartment, and he said that sometimes the place was weird. When I asked him what he meant, he said that he occasionally thought he heard something scurrying around, but that he could never find out what it was, and it gave him the creeps.

"I bet you think I'm crazy, don't you?" he laughed.

"No," I replied. "There are lots of things in this world we can't explain."

Learning to discern the different types of psychic experiences is important to your shamanic practice. It is very easy to become trapped in a subjective cul-de-sac and end up interpreting everything as a psychic encounter. Many times this is born out of the desire to see or make something happen. A calm, determined approach is essential to developing discernment. The best way to avoid becoming silly and gullible is to never try to interpret what you have experienced until you are finished with the experience. Once you leave your trance and return to a normal state of awareness, take a break, then sit back and critically examine what happened. You are not going to have a genuine experience every time, especially in the beginning of your practice. There is simply no need to engage in fanciful self-indulgence. To paraphrase the famous fictional detective, Sherlock Holmes, try to look for everything else it could be before deciding you have experienced the extraordinary. Sometimes it really is just the plumbing or the house settling in the night!

Recently, a group of us were asked to travel to rural Tennessee and examine a church sanctuary where strange, seemingly paranormal events had been occurring, and members of the congregation had become concerned about the possibility of some spirit presence. We were met by the elderly deacon and examined the sanctuary. Once we regrouped outside, we all concluded that, most likely, the energy we felt was that left behind by living people engaged in intense and energetic worship, and no outside presence was intruding. One member of our group reported back to the individual who had asked us to come, and this seemed to resolve the issue.

In another case, while working in Virginia, I went out for a walk after lunch on a very pleasant spring day. Upon returning to my work area, I walked into what could be described as a psychic mist that enveloped me in anger, fear and a strong sense of betrayal. I quickly shielded myself and mentally cleared the room of this psychic debris. About five minutes later, a colleague came over and said, "Boy, did you miss a fight while you were gone!" Apparently, two other colleagues had gotten into a heated argument that was filled with accusations of backstabbing and disloyalty. They had, without knowing it, released a lot of psychic energy into the physical environment, like smoke from a fire. Most humans are psychically messy creatures, and as your awareness evolves, you will be able to detect such energy.

My beloved wife often meditates and chants as a spiritual and therapeutic practice in the evening, especially if I have to work late. I can always tell when she has been doing this by the psychic atmosphere in our home as I enter the door. The sense of peace and serenity is physically palpable.

Some shamanic practitioners develop a relationship with a particular spirit entity, as Lee did with his boys. I have never developed such a formal relationship in my practice. I often feel the presence of my relatives, and

I suppose they watch over me. Often I feel the presence of my beloved maternal grandmother or my paternal great-grandmother. It's up to you to some degree who, how, and if this relationship is sought and acquired.

Once you have opened to their presence, commonplace signs of a spirit presence include the following:

- **A cold spot or the rapid drop of room temperature in a localized part of a room or enclosed area.** Check carefully for open windows, sources of drafts and cracks in the wall before relying on this particular signal.

- **Lights, sounds, smells and/or movement of physical objects that do not seem to have a source or point of origin.** I once investigated a friend's apartment in Charlottesville that was producing strange moaning sounds in the middle of the night. I discovered that the noise originated from the old steam pipes in the basement. It sounded creepy but was not paranormal.

- **Personal dizziness or disorientation with the feeling of weight or pressure on the back or the neck and shoulders.** Leave the area immediately and shield yourself. Upon returning, make sure that the windows are opened, in case of a gas leak or other toxic chemical. If, after all non-paranormal causes have been exhausted, proceed with expelling the entity.

- **Physical contact; being touched, grabbed or struck by an unseen force.** The best course of action is to leave the area and shield yourself. If necessary return and question the entity as to what and why it is acting is such a manner. Often the answer will come in the form of a voice in your head that suddenly pops into your mind.

  Once, while touring a pre-Civil War house that our friends had bought and were restoring near Franklin, Kentucky, I felt several tugs at my arm. Turning around I realized that no one else was near me. I gently asked the spirit who it was and got a child's voice saying something I could not understand. When I reported the incident to my hostess, she replied that she had also encountered the little girl and reminded me that the house was used as a stop on the Underground Railroad. There is no need to react in fear to such situations. This is not a Hollywood movie. Forget what you have been told about ghosts. Most entities, I have found, are just trying to be acknowledged, and common courtesy and kindness are always my first response.

At times when I sense a threat, I instantly construct a psychic barrier around myself with my projected consciousness. There are many ways to do this process, called shielding. Some people wear protective amulets or carry charms on their person. These are fine as a point of focus but remember that they are all essentially props that allow your consciousness to focus in a particular way. I personally use a chant I learned from an African American Christian minister, which goes like this:

I surround myself with the love of God in the name of Jesus Christ!

Through many negative encounters with living and departed entities, this has never failed to protect me as I push my own psychic boundary outward. In order to not retaliate and to return good energy for bad, if I know the source of this energy, I will say:

I commend (name) to the love of God in the name of Jesus Christ! Angels please attend (name).

Again, this has never failed me, although I know that other such methods also work. Above all, you must *not* release fear into the situation. Lee taught me that spirit entities can draw energy from fear, becoming stronger, more physically tangible and hence able to do more damage.

Other non-psychological methods of expelling an evil or negative presence include the use of salt as a barrier, iron and silver as a protective metals and holy or blessed water as a repellent. These are usually employed to clear a physical space of a negative or unwanted presence and are used in conjunction with prayers and incantations, which are used specifically to expel the entity. There was a reason so many old houses had a horseshoe nailed over the door. The whole point in doing any of these magical methods is to restore the physical area to a state of normalcy and to assist those affected in returning to a state of personal equilibrium.

Laughter and ridicule, as well as anger, are another way to put up the psychic barrier to protect yourself against a spirit presence that appears harmful. A spirit entity cannot stand such a psychic onslaught and will withdraw, so keep your fear in check and do what is needed to protect yourself.

As with all things in this life, walking this path is not without risk and it will exact a price from you, so know why you want to be there and what you hope to find. Be prepared to be laughed at, challenged, criticized and shunned by those whom your growing spirituality will threaten. People may say they are with you, but when you do change personally, they will become uneasy, so know why you are doing this practice. The last thing you want to do is to wander aimlessly in this world of the inner mind, for to do so is analogous to wander off into the dark woods without a map or source of light. Above all this is not something with which to play at or pursue as an idle curiosity.

For me, it is a part of a much larger quest for union with the Divine. It has not been an easy path; I have stumbled, fallen and been hurt many times. I have walked in secret and in silence for most of the past thirty years where these matters are concerned; but for me, it has given me a look at a world beyond any I could have imagined and has given me joyous glimpses of an eternity I now long for more than anything else.

CHAPTER EIGHT

I Get More Than I Bargained For

Feel the fear and do it anyway.
> —Susan Jeffers, *Feel the Fear and Do It Anyway*

The human brain is a most unusual instrument of elegant and as yet unknown capacity.
> —Stuart Seaton

IT WAS A BEAUTIFUL, DAY in early November, 1974—the kind that is so beautiful in this part of the Dutch Fork. The leaves seemed to whisper in the steady breeze, which was at once crisp and induced a relaxed, dreamlike state. Lee Gandee was not, however, in a pleasant state when I arrived. He seemed distracted and a bit apprehensive as he let me into his home. He barely spoke and seemed to be watching me carefully. I took my place in the rocker and turned on the recorder. He seemed to barely notice.

"I only have a few questions this morning. . . ." I paused, as Lee's distress was obvious. "Lee, is anything wrong? You seem kind of worried about something."

"I'm just a bit spooked," Lee replied. "The 'boys' have fled the place except Hans Andreas, who's hiding in a back room."

"Hiding from what?"

"Well, I'm not sure I want to tell you. To tell the truth, I'm glad you're here, but I'm a bit afraid for you," he said.

"Okay, Lee, what is this? Are you trying to scare me?"

"No, Jack, I'm not. I have no intention of scaring you. It's just. . . . Have you got your recorder on? If you do turn it off, this is not the time or place."

At this point, I reached down and switched off the recorder.

He then explained that there was an evil spirit in the area that had made its appearance lately in a series of senseless, brutal, crimes. I had heard of the incidents in the local news, but I never assumed that they had any connection to the spirit world. I wondered if Lee was not getting himself worked up over them because he spent so much of his time alone in that old house.

I'd seen other people get themselves to the point of hysteria during a church revival, a séance or a session with an Ouija board. I'd also seen so-called teachers, preachers and other spiritual people, take their disciples, friends and families on an emotional rollercoaster of fear and panic, to the point where they would do anything the charlatan requested, which was mostly a demand for money, sex or obedience.

I was not going to let myself be that gullible, even with someone I liked and trusted. I initially discounted Lee's mood as a sad commentary on aging, as I watched him line his windowsills with salt while chanting prayers of protection. Even after all I'd seen and been through in his presence, I still thought—no, insisted to myself—that I must try to stay as objective as possible. I asked if I could help him, and he shook his head. I sat and smoked a cigarette, feeling slightly annoyed, as he laid a small circle of salt around both of us, chanting all the time.

When he'd finished, he stepped into the circle, sat down and nervously lit his pipe. The scent of his George Washington brand of tobacco began to fill the room. All of a sudden, he sat up straight, as if he'd heard something. I tried to speak, but he shushed me as he listened intently.

I thought to myself, This is ridiculous, I'm going home. As I rose to leave, Lee whispered, "Sit down, please sit down. It's here. What ever you do, don't leave the circle." I sat down, partly out of respect and partly because I glimpsed real fear in his eyes.

At that moment, I felt a sharp thud beneath the floor and a loud noise out in the hallway that led to the kitchen. I told myself that Lee must have concocted a ruse to scare or dazzle me. Then the room's temperature began to drop, in a matter of seconds, from cool to nearly freezing. I looked over at Lee, and he seemed to be in a trance, eyes closed, still chanting softly to himself. I slowly looked around the room. In the corner by the bookcase, I noticed the bottles trembling on the shelf.

As I turned my gaze, I glimpsed a dark, formless mass, about two feet in diameter and four feet in length moving along the wall. I was instantly seized with absolute dread. My blood ran cold as this form moved past the window. Light did not shine through it. Holy shit! I thought; this thing is for real! What the hell am I going to do? I reminded myself not to feed its energy with my fear but folded my hands in prayer and began to softly recite the Lord's Prayer and the 23rd Psalm. I closed my eyes to focus my thoughts on my praying.

"That's it, keep going!" I heard Lee quickly whisper, before returning to his own prayers. I felt the presence draw close to us and was sickened by its foul presence. At one point, I thought I heard it laughing, whispering and then growling. An icy wind began to circle the room, which was incredible since the windows were shut tight. It seemed to have the velocity of an industrial fan spinning 'round like a whirlwind. I kept praying fervently, and in fact, entered a trance myself. I could hear the wind and the noise, but they seemed far away and a strange peace over came me. "Thank you, Lord, thank you for hearing me," I said to myself and to the One who hears all prayers.

At that moment, I heard Lee jump to his feet and yell at the top on his voice, "Get out of here! In the name of the Father, and the Son and the Holy Spirit, I command you to leave the house and return no more!"

What happened next was like something out of some bad horror movie. A piercing shriek, somewhat like a bobcat's scream, was followed by what sounded like claws running across the floor, and the house shook as another loud bang was heard at the back of Lee's bedroom. The room almost instantly returned to it autumn coolness, which seemed warm compared to what it had been just seconds before.

I opened my eyes and saw Lee sitting in his chair across from me, his hands shaking, visibly tired but with a look of relief upon his face. "Thank you," he said softly. "If you had not added your energy when you did, he just might have been able to reach us. Thank you!" We both sat here in silence as the world around us returned to normal. "That was close!" Lee sighed.

"What was that?" I asked, exhausted by this strange experience.

"I'm not quite sure," Lee responded. "The 'boys' say it was a demonic being that has gotten into our world through a hole in the fabric of time and space." He chuckled tiredly. "Say, you look a bit pale! Let's get a cup of coffee, I know I need one."

I stood up and moved to the edge of the salt circle, hesitating to cross it. I also noticed that for all the wind I had felt during those horrible moments, nothing in the room had been disturbed, not even the ashes in the ashtray.

"It's okay," he reassured me. "It's gone! I don't feel it anywhere around here now. Believe me, I would not step out of the circle if I did!"

"Where did it go?" I asked.

"Remember when you felt a calming presence? I remember hearing you thanking God for hearing you in your thoughts. I sensed, at that moment a higher being appeared, intervened and drove it away. Someone up there likes you and watches over you!" he laughed. "I sensed a gentle but powerful female spirit with snow white hair, deep blue eyes and soft gentle hands."

With those words, my eyes welled with tears as I realized that Lee had sensed my beloved, paternal great-grandmother, a healer and the most holy individual I've ever known. Without the slightest trace of self-righteousness or pious pretension, this humble soul could stop an argument by silently walking into the room and just sitting down. Within seconds, her gentle presence filled the room and those who were fighting were now crying in each other's arms. I had never believed in guardian angels until that moment, but if anyone could have and would have intervened to help me at that moment, it would have been her. We adored each other during her life and our bond remains unbreakable to this day. I nodded to Lee through my tears.

"Come on," he repeated. "Let's have that coffee. You need to get yourself together before you try to drive home."

"Am I going to be safe?" I asked nervously. "What if that thing returns?"

"Well. . . ." He got very serious again. "I think it's okay. The 'boys' are out scouting for it, and they say it's gone. But if it does appear, start praying like you did before. . . . I know I will!"

"Lee," I said, as we sat down with the coffee, "what would have happened if it had broken through the circle?"

"I don't know," he replied. "I don't want to think about it."

We sat there in silence, resting, a bit weathered but a lot wiser. "I would not tell anyone about this," he said, as I left for home. "They'll never believe you!" I agreed and have never spoken of it until now.

The Going Gets Even Rougher . . .

"Good morning, Lee!" I said, as I came for a session in mid-May of 1975. We went to his den, as was customary, and sat down. I lit a cigarette and he his pipe. Also in the room was a University of South Carolina (USC) anthropology student whom I came to know as Mike. He was a native of the area and lived near Lee. Mike was a soft-spoken, articulate and pleasant young man and had been studying Powwow with Lee for some time. He had gained Lee's respect for his abilities.

We began to discuss some points from the last session. I remarked to Lee that he had added an open wooden coffin to the eclectic decor of his room. He laughed and said he had purchased it from an auction at an old Odd Fellows' lodge. He thought it made an interesting prop. In the coffin, he had placed a sign reading, "Think about it." We laughed and settled back to talk.

All seemed normal until I began to feel a growing pressure on my shoulders and the back of my neck. I began to feel distracted as Lee was postulating about some point. I silently hoped the recorder was picking up the dialog, as I could barely hear him. It was like listening from inside a tunnel. At one point, I glanced up at the new coffin and observed what appeared to be a partial face looking down at me from it. I thought to myself, This is getting weird; I'd better get the hell out of here right now! I told Lee and Mike that I was feeling suddenly ill and that I'd better go home and get some rest. As I gathered up my things, I remember Lee was very sympathetic. As he showed me to the door, he said he hoped I felt better soon and to give him a call when I did.

I got into the car and started out of the driveway to head home, still feeling the intense pressure on my neck and shoulders. As I proceeded toward the main road, all of a sudden, the car rapidly accelerated and the steering wheel jerked in my hands, appearing to move of its own volition. The car went hurtling down the road at a high rate of speed with the steering wheel operating independently of my attempts to control it, turning corners on screeching tires and taking me heaven knows where.

Stepping on the brakes seemed to have no effect. I became consumed with fear and denial as I repeatedly told myself this just could not be happening. My sense of conventional reality told me there had to be some rational reason for this, but I couldn't think what it might be at the time. I reached for the keys to switch off the motor and the acceleration increased dramatically. By now, I was screaming for it to stop and begging Jesus for help at the top of my lungs, as I raced down a hill at around 70 miles per hour, with a truck looming about 100 yards ahead. Despite my appeals for Divine help, I was too shaken and panicked, as I had never encountered this sort of phenomena outside Lee's presence. I was probably unconsciously empowering my attacker with my hysteria. As the car sailed over a small bridge spanning a creek, the car slowed to a stop, and the intense pressure I had been feeling physically disappeared. I turned off the car and sat gasping for air, trying to calm down and sort out what had happened. Finally, I turned the key in the engine and found it responded normally. I drove straight into Lexington and stopped and the first service station. I told the mechanic about the sudden acceleration and asked him to check the car. He asked if he could drive the car, and I gave him the keys. About 30 minutes later, he came into the waiting area and said he could find nothing out of order and had no explanation for what had just transpired. I paid him and drove slowly home. For the record, the car never again behaved in such a manner for as long as we owned it.

It was on the way home that I began to think that something supernatural had taken place. I checked the tape in the recorder and found that nothing had been recorded, although I had had it on part of the time I was visiting Lee. Whatever I had recorded had been erased. This had never happened before, nor has it happened since the incident with this cassette recorder.

Shortly after that, as my girlfriend and I were taking a late Saturday afternoon nap, we were awakened by a loud voice calling to us. As we roused, a deep, resonant voice announced that he was the spirit of one "Father Matthias." This disembodied voice told us to take Gandee's coffin and our copy of The Long Lost Friend and burn it in Lee's front yard the next Sunday morning. As you might guess, this incident shook both of us to the core, as we cowered in the darkened room. I can still remember my girlfriend saying, "What the hell is going on? Who—what—was that? This is crazy!" I agreed, saying I didn't have a clue, but something had to be done.

At this point, I resolved that this field research had taken a sinister turn and needed to come to an end. For some time, I had been suffering the strain of having to jockey between two conceptions of reality. As fascinating as it was, no project like this was worth the possibility of getting hurt or dealing with phenomena against which I seemed to have no defense. As I entered into this research, I became aware that I was dealing with very different views of reality and life in general. One world was the rational world of college, tests, exams, papers and the social world of girlfriends, parents, jobs and home. It was a world that could be frustrating, but at least it made sense, was predictable and reasonably safe. The other was a world of spirits, witchcraft and invisible forces that could, and did profoundly affect everyday life. It was a world where protective devices and procedures needed to be employed to keep mind and body safe and secure. It was a world where illness was treated as an entity and cured by methods long forgotten by modern science. The strain I experienced had developed as a result of trying to relate a magical view of reality to the rational world without denigrating the magical view of reality or treating it with an attitude of cultural imperialism. Yet to do otherwise was to be accused of losing my scholar's objectivity, of "going native" and so forth. In the magical world, the reliance on rational explanation was treated with contempt, was considered shortsighted.

I balked when I first read Carlos Castaneda's *The Teachings of Don Juan: A Yaqui Way of Knowledge*. As book followed book, I found myself sneering at his loss of objectivity. I remember saying, "Whatever he is doing, it's not anthropology!" As I entered field research myself, I began to understand his struggle and the strain of trying to convey what he had experienced. This was not like doing a survey of kinship or social structure, which were the more typical anthropological or folk study pursuits, but dealt, instead, with the innermost thoughts and feelings of a social group. This deeply personal worldview existed beneath the public persona that a community usually projects. This worldview presented another level of existence. How difficult it must be to come out from such a concept of reality and to try to adapt to the modern scientific perspective required to navigate our modern world! The tenacity of belief systems such as Santeria, modern Powwow and other indigenous traditions of immigrant populations is evidence that such beliefs do not simply fade in the supposed light of science.

"Science is just another way of explaining things," Lee would say. "Not the only way." I finally resolved that until I felt comfortable enough to do otherwise, I would just present what I knew the rational world could manage. As a result, my senior thesis was a historical account of the practice of Hexerei in the Dutch Fork.

The Story Continues . . .

To return to the 1970s, I didn't know what to say to Lee after the terrifying experience with my car, thinking he wouldn't believe me. Worse still, was the thought that he might have had something to do with the incident, although I couldn't think what or why. About two weeks passed, and I resolved to write him and tell him what happened regardless of the consequences to our relationship. I soon received a letter back from Lee, which is excerpted here:

20 June 1975

Dear Jack,

When I got your letter this afternoon I was nonplussed, and then I called my boys [his spirit assistants] and read it to them, and said, "Okay, now which one of you did it?" They protested that they didn't know anything about it, and asked me how I could think that they'd put a visitor and friend of mine through anything so upsetting. "He's not just making it up," I growled. "Somebody did it! Hans Andreas, that would be your idea of having fun—tell me the truth! I know darn good and well that Father Matthai doesn't tell people to burn things in the front yard on Sunday. I've got to find out what happened and who's behind it. . . .

I later learned that Father Matthai was a real historical person. He was a theosophical mystic of the German Pietistic community that settled the Wissahocken Valley in colonial Pennsylvania. He was a pious, holy man, revered and respected in his community. His story can be found in the book The German Pietists of Seventeenth-Century Pennsylvania, by Julius Friedrich Sachse, privately published in 1895 by the author. Only 500 copies of the book were ever printed. Lee owned a copy (#424) that, according to the marks of ownership, was in the Dutch Fork area within two years of its printing. The pages and boards were festooned with hex signs and other magical inscriptions, some of which were faded and indistinguishable with age.

Father Matthai, I learned, was still considered a guardian spirit of a very high order, who watched over believers in matters concerning spirits. His duty was to protect humanity from negative incursions from the spirit. If an evil spirit were to appear in the modern world, Father Matthai would supposedly intervene on behalf of humanity. As described, he seemed to function as some sort of cosmic policeman, restoring order and balance to the realm of humans and spirits.

Lee's extraordinary letter continued. . . .

"Ya always accuse me every time something happens!" Hans Andreas said. "Any spirit could have done it that knows we have a special relationship with him, [this next part is hard to follow, doesn't quite make sense] but doesn't know exactly what it is, or what kind of spirit he [Father Matthai] is. I say some outsider did it!"

No amount of admonition shook their story that when you and Mike [another student of Gandee's] came, they went out and kept out of sight, just in case you might glimpse them and be upset.

I phoned Mike and told his niece to have him call me when he came in, and later one of my friends from Columbia phoned me to check on my plans for the weekend and I told him about the letter. He laughed and said, "I'm surprised he didn't get in touch with you before this." He went on and told me what was in the letter almost word for word; before I had said what you said had happened. He was exultant, and said, "Now do you believe I can do a few things, myself! I've been trying for two years to get through to you, and you always thought I was lying; this was the first chance I ever had to prove what I can do."

"But why on them?" I said.

(I learned that his other college student friend, Mike, had also had a disquieting paranormal experience and was now hesitant to return to Lee's house.)

"I know you don't like Mike because he's got the inside track with me, but why Jack Montgomery?"

"I figured he needed to be shook up." He laughed. "If he's going to write a study of sorcery in South Carolina, he ought to at least know first-hand what it can do to you. The way he was talking, he seemed to think it's all psychological, in the minds of people who are under spells. He had to be blasted loose from that feeling of superiority, anybody can be affected. He had to know that people think they see things, the way he saw the disturbance of light above the coffin, and the face in it, and hear the voice, as he heard the one that said to burn the coffin, to know how real those experiences seem to people who have them. Moreover, he now knows that sorcery can blank out tapes, control automobiles, and the weight and pressure was to let him know some of what a person under a spell suffers."

(This revelation shocked me, as I had not mentioned to Lee in my initial letter this detail, as it didn't seem as important, and I felt I could have been mistaken and left the tape off by accident.)

"Was it one of the Ju-Ju spells you learned in Georgia from the old root doctor?" I asked him.

"I thought you didn't believe he could teach me any," he taunted. "Yes, he taught me."

"Well, I hope you know I don't like it!" I scolded. "Now he'll be afraid to come back, and Mike's not been back either."

"I didn't hurt him, did I?" He laughed. "What did he expect to see at a Hexenmeister's?"

"I don't think he expected to see anything."

"That's what I thought," he said. "I knew you'd not demonstrate anything, and that the boys would stay out of sight. I wanted him to feel a little less sure of himself. He's apt to run up against some black sorcery that could keep him in hot water worse than the weight on his head and neck. I'm not through with him yet. I'm going to really have some fun out of him. If just a half-seen face shakes him up, I'll try to let him see a full-length image next time."

"Your own shape?"

"You know better than that!"

(I learned later that a hex or root doctor will never send out their own shape, as it would identify them and provide a psychic link back to their person. As a result, the mental construct would be disguised in some manner, for protection and for effect.)

"You let him alone!" I said. "That letter—he's just not able to stand the strain. I'm going to phone Mike and find out if he saw you, and if you scared him till he's not coming back, you know what I told you."

"I don't think he saw anything or felt anything," he said. "You have too many barriers around him, and he's got power enough to keep his head on straight even if he should see anything—he'd know what it was."

"Mike's met with the spirit out at Nazareth," I said. "Jack's not ever seen anything more than an ordinary ghost."

"Did you think of that when you invited him over there?" He laughed. "If he'd seen Mike's black leopard who walks like a man and talks to your boys, and Snakebird's Indian god that looks like a six-foot woodpecker, what would you have told him?"

"I'd have told him they were illusions," I said, "Mere hallucinations."

"Then tell him the face in the coffin was an illusion," he chuckled, "and the weight he felt."

"Nothing but a psychological state."

"He'd better say that in his thesis anyhow."

"You could have caused him to get killed if he'd rammed that truck."

"I could, but I wasn't going to. I'm not going to hurt your friends. I just wanted him to get good and scared, so he'd know how a person feels when he's controlled by sorcery."

"You've had your fun now. You've got to let him alone."

"Who tells you you have got to do anything?" he chuckled. "I'm going to show him a lot more things. I won't hurt him, just shake him up so he'll write his thesis with clearer realization of what he's talking about."

"I'm warning you, you'd better not play around with Father Matthai. Imitating his voice was not too smart."

"I said my name was Matthias," he laughed. "That's not the same name."

"I going to warn him you'll still be plaguing him," I said.

"Yeah, I want him to know it!" He chuckled. "Then what he sees and experiences won't scare him so, merely leave him dumbfounded."

"If you hurt him, you're going to answer to me!"

"I said I wasn't going to hurt him," he said. "I'm just going to give him something to write about in his thesis."

Well, that's the story. A man I never took seriously before caused it all because he was bored, and came over here astrally, and thought it would be fun to shake you up. There are a lot of such jokers around and plenty who are not so well disposed and not friends of mine. I stay flexible and no matter what I see, I try not to lose my cool. You do the same. If you feel anything such as the weight, run water over your hands and arms and wash your face, if you can't take a shower, and you'll be all right.

And carry a silver coin, and if it turns black, bathe in rosemary water and rue, and scour the coin bright with charcoal or rotten brick powder. This man sleeps till 3 A.M. and does his work between then and sunrise. If anything hits you right after 3:00 A.M., make a note of it; and you'll notice things happening to you in runs of threes as long as he's having fun with you. He's apt to make your dream life pretty wild and foul up your sex life. He saw your girlfriend when he went to tell you what to tell me to do with the coffin, and he wants her for himself. I'm just afraid he'll louse things up between you and try to barge in and take her from you. So no matter how odd or erratic she acts for a while, don't let any quarrel get started. This guy is not a black witch, and he's not a bad guy, but he's not entirely scrupulous."

At this point, the letter continues on some other matters and later returns to the incident, saying that Mike, too, had sensed something going on and was uneasy, but he did not experience the types of things I had described. At the conclusion of the letter, Lee reminded me not to be upset with whatever I see or hear. He added:

I'd think that as much as you've seen and heard about, you'd be even better able to handle other realities."

I believe he was referring to my studies in conjure and Eastern religions. Finally, he advised,

You simply can't give in to things like that, or you'll be climbing the walls or looking out through the bars at the Bull Street landscape [referring to the South Carolina state mental hospital in Columbia]. If you'd only told me you saw the face, I'd have told you to go to the bathroom and wash your face and hands. If you're scared to come back, at least write or phone me, for I certainly don't want to lose touch with you.

Cordially, Lee

About a week later, an editor for Prentice Hall (the publisher for Lee's book, *Strange Experience: The Secrets of a Hexenmeister: How to Employ the Hex Signs and Spoken Spells of Rural American Folk Magic*), who wishes to remain anonymous, sent me a letter printed on the company letterhead. Apparently, Lee had contacted his editor, told him my story and asked him to vouch for him. The letter read as follows:

25 June 1975

Dear Mr. Montgomery,

My good friend Lee R. Gandee wrote me of your disquieting experiences with his coffin, your car, and later the voice in the night. Lee felt you were pretty wrought up, and rightly so, but following your letter to him, I'd say he's solved the mystery to his satisfaction and mine, and hopefully yours. Suffice it to say that Lee has a good friend who delights in playing psychic tricks of quite sophisticated scope. He told me in a letter exactly how my basement looked and described a painting over the fireplace—here in Jersey! After Lee's friend did a magic ritual to investigate a matter of interest to him in Tenafly, my hometown, a lady who was the object of his curiosity discovered tracks of a cat and a snake in the January snow by her home—both animals which Lee's friend said he sent to find out for him.

Lee's friend has gotten some powerful learning from a Georgia Root-Doctor, and while he does have a grand fondness for practical jokes, his head's in the right place and his heart a good one. Lee and I would still be doubting his powers if he hadn't related the coffin-burning instructions you "heard" before Lee had told him of your letter. Lee too is a man of good heart, and I can assure you, you have nothing to fear from him. As for his friend, he was merely trying to show you that any investigation into magic is bound to raise some surprises for you, and he wanted to give you a taste of what you might expect to happen once you began your researches. (This was all done in a spirit of gleeful, disinterested prankishness, but it's well to think what you'd encounter if you were faced with someone with real hostility.) Lee better than anyone can tell you how to protect yourself from such influences, and I can tell you step one is not to fear anything. You must able to test an apparition or voice as you would

a used car dealer, and without the courage of your convictions, you are
powerless. But Lee's friend is not evil, however mischievous, and neither
he nor Lee would think of doing you the least harm. And with the power
I have at my command, I declare you protected, and so you are. But you
must be ready to ask the Devil why he wears his hooves that way, and
always ask why when a voice tells you to do anything. And just because the
spirit is real, what it says may not be. You are the equal of any discarnate
because you have a body to boot, and I do hope you can resume pleasant
conversation with Lee, who's one of the sanest and genuinely benevolent
guys I've ever known, and as I hope to be. So if any spirit threatens you,
tell it it'd better clear things with Old ———— first. "Have your fears
and have your fun, and you learn, no harm's been done."

Peace and good wishes. . . .

After reading the letters, I sat wondering to myself how any of this
could be true. Was this some sort of elaborate mind game or scheme to
convince me of his supposed powers and abilities? I was well aware from
my other fieldwork that sometimes such charismatic people will exploit
odd, yet natural phenomena to win over their followers' credibility. What
if he was telling the truth as he knew it? What if he himself was being
psychologically exploited by a person I will call "Dwayne"? I realized that
at times, in encounters like these, elaborate mind games are employed by
both sides in an attempt to gain recognition and power. To some degree,
Lee had allowed the incident in the orchard, where his anger had magically
destroyed everything in it. Lee's actions may have inadvertently harmed the
individual who had insulted and verbally abused him. Perhaps Lee acted in
this way to remain unchallenged and to enhance his status as a powerful,
magical person in the community.

I showed the both letters to my senior advisor in the Department of
Religious Studies at the University of South Carolina. I asked him whether
he thought I should continue this project or stop and use what I had to
this point. He was curious, sympathetic and concerned for me, but thought
that if I believed I could manage what happened, I should continue the
research.

I Achieve an Odd Notoriety

Oddly enough, this incident and my reporting it to faculty gave me an
odd notoriety and sometimes unwelcome reputation in the department. I
became a curiosity to people, who would stop me and secretly confide their
own paranormal experiences to me. Strange folks would approach me on
campus asking my advice on occult matters. I uniformly refused to involve
myself and insisted that this was an academic pursuit. I was asked to lecture
at several religious studies and anthropology classes on my fieldwork. Once,
attending a public lecture on traditional healing and speaking up during the
question and answer period, I was approached by a local newspaper on my
topic. I gave what I thought was a carefully worded account of my academic
interest, only to have my statements misquoted. I found myself presented
as a local eccentric, to say the least. I should have known better, but youth
and egotism ruled the day, to my sincere regret.

Recently, as my wife and I were visiting New Orleans, we chanced to
have a conversation with a Voodoo priest in a local museum. As we talked,
he remarked that in the contemporary magical worldview, there are three
types of people: those who are genuinely sincere; those who are looking
for someone to follow, to answer all their personal issues and lead them
spiritually by the hand; and those who are charismatic, knowledgeable but
personally insecure. The Voodoo priest went on to say that insecure individuals are frequently led by fragile and ego-driven ambition down a spiraling
path, to their detriment and the detriment of others who are equally insecure. These followers often want someone to lead them to the "la-la land"
of feel-good, no self-responsibility spirituality. I agreed, as during the past
thirty years, I have seen this scenario played out many times in a variety of
spiritual groups ranging from evangelical Christians to Eastern guru followers to Wiccan covens. The group dynamics and disappointing results are the
same. It is incredibly hard to resist the enchantment that comes with having
people turn to you spiritually, especially if you have never felt that sort of
acceptance before, but it is an enchantment nonetheless. Public acclaim is a
powerful narcotic and its addictive hold is very hard to shake.

Over the years, I have been asked many times to be someone's spiritual
guide or teacher. I always respectfully decline but offer to send them resources

for their own search. I can always tell the ones who will do nothing with my offer, as I won't allow them to surrender their discrimination and self-responsibility. Any journey of the spirit that will lead you to a direct experience of the Divine is a solitary one, despite what dogmas and doctrines may assert. Spiritual growth is not unlike the transitions from childhood to adolescence to adulthood. Beyond the early stages, one's real spiritual growth is not always safe, easy or anyone else's responsibility. Even the magical path, with all its miraculous events, is only a glimpse, a way of opening the heart and mind to the infinite possibilities of a direct, mystical encounter with the Divine. The only thing a responsible teacher should do is to show you the ways they have learned and point you in the direction they believe might take you where you want to go. It has always fascinated me how willing people are to throw their caution and good sense to the wind and follow someone who offers them a quick-and-easy way to spiritual growth. It must be like the lure and enchantment of get-rich-quick schemes or gambling. It must be the unwillingness to delay one's rewards in order to acquire them along with the wisdom to manage them properly.

Facing Unexpected Challenges

On several occasions as I lectured to USC classes on my field research, I sometimes found myself facing people who I learned were notable figures in the local occult community. One day, a tall Caucasian man, who was known locally to be a Huna or Hawaiian priest, came to one of my talks, carrying a large, carved walking stick. With him was a retinue of young ladies, all of whom I was told were his personal sex-slaves. Thinking this could only be the one such individual I'd heard about, I greeted him by name as I passed by, which startled him. He was very respectful of my talk and shook my hand as he left. I soon found myself among people I had never met before, but who were known in local occult circles. I thought, perhaps, these folks came to see if I knew what I was talking about. I suppose they came to "check me out," to verify my authenticity—and probably "checking out the competition." Most seemed simply curious but sometimes these encounters took on a bizarre ambience.

On another day, I came to a Religious Studies class and was met at the door by the professor, who informed me that another so-called Huna had come to class to do "psychic battle" with me. I walked in, nodded and smiled to the only unfamiliar face in the class and took a seat in front of him. During the lecture, I could hear him physically straining and quietly chanting and making a serious effort to make some impression upon me. I remained calm and psychically shielded myself as Lee had taught me. I took my class notes as usual, thinking how stupid this whole affair had become. After about a half hour of apparently unsuccessful effort, he cried out and bolted from the classroom. The professor stared with wide-eyed amazement at me. I smiled, shrugged my shoulders and returned to my notes.

I was later informed by the professor that this individual had burst into his office crying and asking to be released from my spell. I denied placing any spell and suggested that the boy had other issues that needed professional attention. The local occult community of Columbia, South Carolina, in 1975 appeared to be the year that a plethora of white, Anglo-Saxon males aspired to be traditional Hawaiian shamans. It must have been our warm weather, excellent seafood and proximity to the ocean! At times, the atmosphere was circus-like, much to my dismay, as I saw my work becoming trivialized by these attention-seekers.

After another guest lecture to a religious studies class, I was gathering my things when a young, pretty African American student asked if we could speak in private. As we sat in the empty room, she relayed the sad story of her uncle, who, once an intelligent and successful man of robust health, had fallen under the spell of a root doctor's curse and now lay in the local veteran's hospital—a withdrawn, shriveled shadow of his former self. Both physicians and clergy had been consulted but failed to effect a cure for his condition. She asked me if I could please help him. I apologized, saying that I was not sure he would respond to me, partly because I was white, and secondly that I was not from the Sumter area. In short, I felt that he would not know or trust me, and therefore, I would not be effective. I suggested that she find a root doctor from the Sumter area to come in and remove the curse. Looking dejected, she thanked me and left. I felt bad that I didn't try in some way to help, but I also didn't want to expand my occult reputation any further than it had already spread. Several months later, I ran into the same young woman on campus and inquired after her uncle, only to be informed that he had passed away. I remember feeling really guilty about that incident for a long time afterward. I resolved not to make that mistake again. If someone asked me to lay hands or pray over them or their loved ones, I would do it. Let people think what they will, my conscience is clear.

After much soul-searching and encouragement from my professors, I decided to return to the field research and went to Lee Gandee's house again. Lee began to instruct me in methods of protecting myself against any further attempts by Dwayne to "have some fun" out of me. In reality, I employed every technique and began to treat the things I learned and events that happened in and around this project as if they were valid. As I told my college advisor, "If nothing else, it makes me feel more secure, and I can concentrate on what I'm supposed to be doing on this project."

An Epilogue of Sorts . . .

About a year later, I went to visit Lee at his new lodgings in West Columbia. As I entered the kitchen, there sat a man in his late twenties at the table, drinking a beer at three in the afternoon. Somehow, I just knew it was the young root doctor who had given me such a scare, so I addressed him with a cheery "Hello, Dwayne. That was a pretty mean trick you played on me back there."

"Dwayne" looked up and said, "Well, I thought you were a little too pompous and needed to be taught a lesson."

"A bit of a dangerous lesson," I responded.

"You weren't in any danger," he replied. "If I had wanted to hurt you, you wouldn't have survived."

"Understood!" I replied and went into the other room to find Lee.

I never saw or spoke to Dwayne again. Lee indicated that Dwayne had been using drugs and alcohol, and as a result, had lost his powers. It was quite well known that alcohol and drugs thwarted, or at least significantly hindered, any ability to focus or employ one's psychic abilities. If you wished to do magic, you needed to be free of any foreign substance and in good mental health. Dwayne, as Lee later noted, eventually reaped the results of his negative magical behaviors by succumbing to alcohol. To my knowledge, even though some other odd things happened during this period of my field research, I could never attribute anything else directly to Dwayne.

At this point in time, at this distance from those events, it's difficult to analyze with absolute certainty these and the other unusual events I encountered. It is important to note that once someone psychologically enters into what I call the magical mindset of the shaman, perception and interpretation of events becomes enhanced. One perceives things that are, for the most part, invisible to others immersed in everyday consciousness. For example, two individuals will witness a certain event—a movement in the grass during a moonlit night. One person will just see light and shadows, while the person in the shamanic mindset will be more open to the subtle expressions and see an entity moving through the grass, drawing inferences that would otherwise be ignored.

This is not to say that either perception is incorrect or a delusion of some sort. I have observed people in church, absorbed in prayer and meditation and perceiving a communication with a Divine source. Yet, in the same church, facing the same physical stimulus, other people sit, simply observing the space around them, with no such direct spiritual encounter. When asked if they have experienced anything, they will sometimes indicate that they have enjoyed the atmosphere, but that is all. No message, no rapture, no answer or sign. Is one of these people deluded and the other not? Clearly, our culture generally recognizes and accepts these differences in perception only within certain officially recognized contexts. I would assert, therefore, that within the context of cultures that officially recognize the shamanic magical mindset, to experience unusual events and respond to them accordingly is appropriate, normal and not a delusion or hallucination.

It appears that what we experience, how we experience it and what each of us, as individuals, consider normal is, to some degree, determined by our social enculturation. We experience what we expect to experience without being aware that we have been programmed to ignore everything else. If we catch a glimpse of something beyond our expectations, we find that experience psychologically and even physically disturbing and may experience emotional trauma. The most commonly recognized form of these phenomena occurs when an average person encounters some visual or auditory manifestation of the paranormal, such as glimpsing a ghost or hearing a disembodied voice. Modern people who have this sort of experience will typically go to great lengths to restore their regular state of awareness as quickly as possible. They will usually dismiss the experience as a hallucination or a case of mistaken identification. They may then seek confirmation from those they trust that what they experienced could not have been real. Finally, they often seek to avoid situations they perceive as having brought the experience about—such as steering clear of a house known to be haunted. People who frequently have these unusual experiences are often considered mentally unbalanced and are to be socially avoided. We do not normally accept those into our social groups who do not see the world as we do. This rejection becomes a very effective method of social control, as we circle our wagons in defensively against anything that might threaten our sense of control.

Most of us have been taught to ignore and not acknowledge the appearance of a spirit world. The traditional shaman or religious mystic has learned to open his or her perception to include it, in a controlled manner, and accept the experience. To be an effective mystic or shaman from a typically scientific rationalistic society, one must consciously resist cultural training that insists that such things do not happen. One must slowly and carefully learn to open one's awareness to this additional aspect of reality and accept the experience when it occurs. This is a slow, deliberate learning process and a skill that usually takes many years to master.

Endings and Beginnings

It was December of 1976, and I graduated college. As the months rolled by, Lee and I began to drift away from each other as our lives took different directions. I would call on him from time to time, and our conversations were mostly on mundane topics. It was clear that our spiritual connection had run its course. It all happened in a very natural and friendly manner.

During our last meetings, I found myself, at the request of a mutual friend, gently scolding him about the careless way he was pursuing his now openly gay lifestyle. I had no objection to his being gay. I have always believed that gay people are simply another expression of the Divine's infinite love, and I have always believed that the Divine made no mistakes in our creation. What concerned everyone who knew and loved Lee was that some of the people he was associating with were a threat to his health and personal safety. I remember seeing him in his living room, slumped in a chair, staring childlike at the floor, agreeing with my concern and acknowledging the danger in which he was placing himself.

"You have always been straight with me," he said. "I do appreciate your concern for me, and I know you've never judged me."

"I know you, Lee," I replied. "You are a good and decent person, and I will always care about you, no matter what. Just be good to yourself." He nodded.

After that final meeting, I would often hear gossip about him and occasionally read some letter-to-the editor that he had written in the local newspaper, but life just moved on for both of us.

I left Columbia in 1978 to attend graduate school at the University of Virginia. I heard no more of or from Lee until I learned of his death. As I said before, a teacher can only point the way; the relationship of teacher and student should be transitory. The journey and practice of Powwow had, in reality only just begun for me. It led me to other teachers and experiences, which I will share with you in the next few chapters.

CHAPTER NINE

The Legacy Continues . . .

The glorious gifts of the gods are not to be cast aside.

—Homer, *The Iliad*

From the Gods, to the earth, to man,
From man, to the earth, to the Gods
A gift for a gift.

—Scandinavian/Germanic offering invocation

Powwow on the Web!

While surfing the web one day, I came across a review of Lee Gandee's book (now out of print), *Strange Experience: The Secrets of a Hexenmeister: How to Employ the Hex Signs and Spoken Spells of Rural American Folk Magic,* on Amazon.com. I proceeded to write a review of the title. To my surprise, I was soon contacted by a man asking me if I had really met Lee and studied with him in the past. He indicated that he ran an online chat room devoted to the modern day study of Powwow and Lee's book. He invited me to join their discussions, which I did. The online group is on Yahoo, under "PA Dutch Wiccans and Powwows." To my astonishment, there existed a well-organized group of people who read and study traditional Powwow. I became acquainted with "Oracle" and his wife "Rose." After many online conversations, I decided to take a detour from a business trip in January 2003 to visit Oracle and Rose. The following conversations were recorded on January 28, 2003, in southern Pennsylvania, at their home. They asked me not to include their real names for fear of reaction from their small-town community. They live in a spacious but modest dwelling with their two children. Oracle and Rose are in their early thirties and maintain a lovely,

well-appointed home. Their children were well-behaved, and Oracle and
Rose were gracious hosts and excellent cooks. Here are some segments of
our conversations.

Working with the Spirit World

Rose: Tell him the bird story.

Oracle: My mom was going with friends to visit a medium who used a
         Ouija board as a vehicle. She wanted to contact her grandmother.
         Before she left, she also asked her second husband if there was
         anyone he wished to contact. He told her that his mother used to
         talk to the birds and receive messages from the spirit world. He
         wanted my Mom to ask her what did the birds say to her when
         they used to talk to her.

            My mom went to the medium and got through to the spirit
         world. She could not reach her mother-in-law, and the spirits said
         she could not contact my great-grandmother because "she was
         elevated." Do you know what that means?

Jack: Yeah, okay, to be elevated gets into the Hex worldview of our
         reality existing in multiple dimensions, like the layers of an onion.
         Most mediums can only make contact with the world right next
         to our own. Spirits can be on one level after they have just passed
         over, and they can exist there for eons. If they or their consciousness
         continues to evolve, they will move into much more subtle realms
         and become elevated. That was according to Lee [Gandee].

Rose: And what are those realms like? I guess nobody knows.

Jack: Not according to the spirits we can reach in the next realm to this
         one. Occasionally you can supposedly get to the elevated levels, and
         they will answer you, but generally you are just picking up spirits
         that are operating mentally on the same level as when they had a
         physical form coexistent to our own.

Rose: Okay, sort of like the John Edwards thing where they come knock-
         ing.

Jack: I once asked Lee about what spirits told him of heaven and the life eternal and he replied, "They don't know about that! They are often just as confused as we are. They are just on the next level of existence." Spirits can move beyond the realms you and I currently exist within, and many are taking their time, like wandering travelers and are just riding around, enjoying themselves, wandering in and out of life on our plane of existence. The idea is that you live at multiple levels of existence at the same time. We are living in this dimension at the same time we exist in other dimensions. Lee had this term he would use for a spirit who could move between different levels of existence. He called it an "ultra-terrestrial." I have never found another definition of that word, and as far I knew then and now, it is a made-up word. As we exist across these multiple dimensions, we focus our consciousness at any one time into a single dimension and that dimension appears real to us at that time. This is usually that dimension where we feel the most solid, like the one we are focused in right now. This makes us appear to have "incarnated" into a single plane of existence. We all are, as Lee would say, "moving energy" or "embodied consciousness" and the spirit world next to this one is a bit less solid, yet it feels solid to you. Finally, as we move through the layers, we come to a state where we are pure thought, undifferentiated consciousness, like a huge deep pool of essence. You are always, a projection of this eternal consciousness—that is the only thing that truly exists within you and that does not change. Everything else is the result of being physically embodied and is therefore subject to change.

Rose: But it seems that on this plane there is pain and suffering. Is there any of that on the other plane?

Jack: Sure!

Rose: But you hear that everything is supposed to be so wonderful over there. This is what I don't understand. You say they [spirits] hang around you; they get into the car. . . .

Jack: They usually are working out things they have not resolved here.

Rose: *[laughing]* Oh! I'm going to be stuck here for good!

Jack: Not necessarily! I asked Lee how long a spirit stays around the next plane. He said, "As long as they need to." With a multidimensional self, like when you dream, you are often in one of those parallel universes, dimensions. I don't mean the kinds of dreams where your consciousness is just blowing off steam, the crap you've dealt with, your closet of anxieties. I'm talking about the other, more intense kind of dreams, that are crystal clear, where you more fully experience the events in that so-called dream. This is, according to Lee, a visit to another universe or plane of existence.

Rose: He [nodding toward Oracle] has those all the time.

Oracle: Yeah! But let me finish the story. My mom asked to speak with the mother of her second husband. A spirit came forth saying that she was that spirit. My mother asked the spirit the question, "What did the birds tell to you when you spoke to them?" The answer to all these questions came back in German and this woman, in life, spoke only German.

Jack: When did she live?

Oracle: I know she was in her twenties and thirties during the rise of Nazi Germany. That was the reason they left.

Jack: So she was born around the turn of the century.

Oracle: Yeah! They wanted to leave, as the Nazis were trying to recruit their son for the Nazi youth, so they saw the handwriting on the wall. Maybe she foresaw what was coming in a magical work.

Jack: Did she practice?

Oracle: I don't know for sure. I know that when my mom returned to her husband that night, she told him she'd gotten a message, but she'd have to get it translated from the German. When he opened the paper containing the two words in German, he turned white as a sheet. The words were "kleine Geheimnisse" and that was what his mother used to tell him the birds would tell her, "small secrets."

Rose: It scared Oracle's mother to the point that she has a gift but will not use it. It's very sad!

Oracle: She sat before us and proclaimed . . . "If I wanted to do that stuff,

I could and I'm good at it." She's just scared to do it.

Jack: For a lot of folks, magic is very threatening because it rattles their reality grid.

Oracle: It sure does. That's one of the things that led me to my magical name, Oracle, which means a seer. Not so much that I am clairvoyant or anything like that, but I have had those experiences.

Jack: Did you have them as a child?

Oracle: Yeah! The first one I remember was when I was sleepwalking and ran into my "Pop-pop" [paternal grandfather]. I asked him, "What are you doing here?" He told me everything was all right and to go back to sleep. I knew my dad had been in a car wreck and Pop-Pop was trying to get to him. My dad was indeed in a car wreck on one of the bridges and almost died. I remember visiting him in the hospital.

Jack: You said your family had a background in all of this. Can you explain what you meant?

Oracle: They did. My mother's grandmother was a "wise woman." They said she was involved in politics, but it was more than that. She would sit at the bar, and say something like "God's going to get him for that!" Next thing you knew, that person turned up dead. This woman would make that call and boom, it happened. I don't know how you would read that—as a coincidence or what. . . .

Jack: But it happened repeatedly?

Oracle: Yeah! My mom said that when she'd say it, everyone would get nervous.

Jack: It would make me nervous. [Laughter]

Oracle: She was big on herbal remedies and poultices. She used a potato poultice. . . .

Rose: My mom used the mustard and potato poultices.

Oracle: Yeah! The best one was to put the mustard in the bathwater and put the baby in it—

Rose: —for the fever seizures, to bring the fever down. We used it twice for our daughter, who had them when she was cutting molars two days before her second birthday. My mother-in-law had her and took her to the hospital. After we got her home, we thought we had the fever down, and five minutes later she was seizing again. I was five months pregnant, and I said, "That's it!" We did it here and it worked. My mother told us what to do. She knew the fever chant, the colic chant. . . .

Jack: What did she do for the colic?

Rose: My great-grandmother used to put the baby's t-shirt on a broom handle and run up and down the alleyway with some kind of chant. My grandmother won't talk about it, and my mother won't either, so I guess it's lost. It's a shame. You know, I took my name, Rose, because she grew roses.

Jack: So both of you have the family connection.

Oracle: Yeah, both of us. My grandmother used to go into the woods to gather materials for the poultices and for us to take. When she used to do Braucherei or what they call Powwow, she would do it with a group of people in a healing circle.

Jack: Do you know how many people were involved?

Oracle: I don't know; it could have been around ten or even more. I will have to ask my mom, but it often was a large gathering. Something like a prayer meeting. . . . They would gather and do their chanting and their work, using the Christian divinity, and away they'd go. Most times the person got better unless it was God's time to take them.

Rose: My grandmother did it with the Christian divinity too. She had the guardian, Mary, up there. Mary was the center; Mary had roses in front of her all the time [referring to a home altar].

Oracle: Did your great-grandmother ever play with a Ouija board?

Rose: Not that I know of. . . .

Oracle: Mine did!

Rose: I know she did have a visitation from my great-grandfather after he died. He sat on the end of her bed and told her everything was all right and not to worry.

Oracle: He spoke to her? Did she see his apparition?

Rose: She said she felt him sitting on the bed.

Jack: I remember my grandmother telling me how they would keep the corpse in the house for three days. Lee said that they did that first to make sure you were dead and second to let the spirit regain consciousness and see that it was dead. Apparently many spirits do not realize they are dead right away.

Rose: Yeah! They used to lay you out right in the living room. In our area, they used to take the hearse by the house so the person would see it and realize their condition, but they don't do that any more. My father told me they did it with my great-grandmother.

Oracle: It's interesting that in Judaism, they try to bury them before sundown the next day.

Rose: They don't embalm them, and I guess it would be unpleasant to wait too long.

Oracle: You've got to wonder, there must be a lot of good Jewish ghosts in the graveyard wondering what the heck is going on. *[Laughter]*

Jack: Of course, they [Jews] have their own mystical tradition called the Kabbalah.

Rose: A friend of ours is into the Kabbalah.

Oracle: She has a large garden of cinquefoil (five-finger grass). They always have money. . . . I was reading in the Herr book about the magic wish bone and feeding it with the mullein root. You put it in oil or whiskey.

Jack: I remember asking Lee why you put a root in whiskey and he would say, "'Cause spirits like whiskey!" And I asked him, "Can they taste it?" He said that they could taste the essence of it, and they like it as they did when they lived on this plane. Fairies also like whiskey, and I asked him if you could go out after and drink an offering you had left for them the next morning. He replied, "You'd better not! You'd better just pour it out on the ground."

Oracle: If you think about it, in the attempts to reconstruct German hea-
         thenism, the favored drink of the German pantheon is mead (honey
         wine). They [deities] also like beer and ale. We make offerings of
         beer and ale in our rituals. The next morning we always go down
         and pour it out under a tree in the front yard.

Rose: That tree has grown like, three feet since we've been feeding it. It's
         my "Blessing Tree." It gets a lot of alcohol!

Oracle: It's a happy tree! *[Laughter]*

Rose: It is a happy tree! Every year we decorate it more and more for
         Christmas.

Oracle: There is a German method of doing that [disposing of a libation/
         offering]. It's an acknowledgement also used in Scandinavia. When
         you pour out your libation overnight, you make the "gebo" rune,
         which symbolizes balance, equilibrium. . . . It also has an invocation
         that goes:

         "From the Gods, to the earth, to man,
         From man, to the earth, to the Gods,
         A gift for a gift."

And then make the gebo over the offering.

Jack: That has a similar pattern to a chant for a healing: "From the bone,
         to the muscle, from the flesh to the skin. . . ."

Oracle: This was a northern German practice. They were influenced by the
         Scandinavian cultures. I don't know if it would have been the same
         in southern Germany.

Rose: My grandmother was from southern Germany, from the old Austro-
         Hungarian Empire. They lived in what was Austria. She was born in
         1901, and the family emigrated in 1903. They settled in Philadelphia
         and are there to this day. We moved to the country to try to get
         away from the crime and give our kids a better chance.

   We then went on to talk about other magical aspects and practices.
Our backgrounds in Powwow were different, so it was interesting to share
ideas.

Spirits and Spell Casting

Oracle: I do have the power to communicate with the spirit world while in a lucid dream state. I appear to be disconnected enough from the regular world that they can come through. I get this from my mother's side of the family. It has been very useful to us in the past. [To Rose] Tell him about Grandmother and Michelle [their four-year-old daughter].

Rose: About three years ago, we were trying for a baby. I wanted to be pregnant so bad. We decided to have a handfasting one Beltane [May Day]. We were already married, but we wanted to do this in the hope that it would bless us with a baby. His mother attended; we all had a great time and everything was beautiful. In the meantime, however, Oracle had had one of those dreams several weeks before; that his grandmother came to him, and she had a little girl with her. She asked him if the child could stay and he told her yes. I got pregnant soon after. . . . We had the baby blessed on the following Beltane. Quite a story, huh?

Oracle: This was one of those dreams that are more real than a regular dream.

Rose: When our daughter was eighteen months old, I came in one afternoon and she's standing in the crib just waving at something. I asked her "Who are you waving to, Michelle?"

"'Bye," she said. I repeated my question and she replied, "Bob, Bob!" She didn't know any "Bob" and I didn't either, until I realized later that Oracle's father used to be called Bob.

Jack: Is he alive?

Oracle: No, he died several years before Michelle was born.

Rose: Also, when we moved into this home, we inherited a lot of Oracle's grandmother's furniture. When it came into the house, she came with it.

Jack: How so?

Oracle: It was her furniture. The furniture was her prized possession. She's here with us today. We sense her presence quite often. It's very comforting.

Jack: Lee used to say that spirits will congregate in the least occupied part of a house. We apparently interfere with their energy, as we are a lot more tangible than they are. This is the part of Hexerei that fascinates me, but you have to watch it. It has an addictive quality.

Rose: I know. You feel that you want to communicate all the time.

Jack: Yep! I have known people who submerged themselves to the point where they were seeing spirits all the time. I really don't want to see them all the time! *[Laughter]* I want to be able to turn it on and off.

Oracle: Yes, I know what you mean. I want the knowledge and am able to use it but keep it on a "need to know" basis.

Jack: Lee told me of a woman he knew who reached the point she could not tell the living from the dead.

Oracle and Rose: *[in unison]* That's not good!

Rose: That's really unhealthy. I wouldn't want to live like that.

Jack: They eventually had to put her in a facility.

Rose: I guess so, she was nuts! *[Laughter]*

Jack: To the average world, absolutely. Lee said she would speak to and relay messages from people he had known in his past. She would relay details she just could not have known, as she was not around these people or even knew them. Medium-ship is a fine line and one to be approached with care.

Oracle: That's for certain. There must be a proper balance, and you must stay connected to the reality you currently inhabit.

Soon we began exchanging stories of healing practices we had used or heard about. Oracle and Rose had been taught by their families while I had learned most of mine from Lee.

Healing Practices

Jack: Lee and some other Hexes always used the thumb as a focal point with the fist turned downward and pointed at the floor when they performed a healing. Are you familiar with this hand posture? Do you know the origin of this practice?

Oracle: Speaking of the old German, the thumb is associated with Wotan. I also use my thumb in a healing, and I believe in doing so, I am channeling the healing power of Wotan through my thumb. I am assuming then that if you used your dominant hand to heal, you'd use the other to hex. I have never had cause to do the negative, but I can also see why the left/right, good/bad symbolism would be so easy for the Christians to accept.

Jack: It was already a part of their culture.

Oracle: Right! We may never know exactly how they used it before Christianity came, but if you read Tacitus's *Germania*, he talks about the worship of trees.

Jack: Have you ever seen a tree augured? [Auguring is a form of spell-casting involving the placement of a written spell often combined with items to work the sympathetic magic and to personalize the spell.]

Oracle: No, but I gave my cousin a ritual for her child's croup. She's a Christian, so I gave her that version so she'd be comfortable with it. She is in the family line to know this stuff. The ticket [written spell] was placed and sealed in the hole she bored into the tree. It worked. Would you call that a *Himmelsbrief*?

Jack: Not necessarily. A ticket is for variety of purposes, and a *Himmelsbrief* is strictly a protective device. As early as the Civil War and even in the first and second World Wars, mothers would give their sons a *Himmelsbrief* to wear to protect them. Writing was considered sacred, if not magical, as a lot of folks couldn't do it. For example, up in Appalachia, a lot of people could not write, but they could make symbols—they could create on paper what they needed to have happen.

Oracle: Would this be like the *anhangsel* that Lee spoke about?

Jack: The *anhangsel* was a protective device created for the person, usually at birth and worn on the person. Often it was stamped on metal, like a military dog-tag.

Oracle: I wonder if runes could have been used. You know, the Pennsylvania Dutch probably would not have been impressed with just words, but if they saw runes, they might believe that it was some sort of heavy magic. Have you ever seen an *anhangsel*?

Jack: Only in a book.

At this point, Rose called us in for a delicious dinner. After dinner, we discussed Karl Herr's book, *Hex and Spellwork: The Magical Practices of the Pennsylvania Dutch*.

Rose: I read this book right after New Year's Eve in about two hours and just pored through it. It talked about making a throw stick . . . fire walkers . . . all of it.

Jack: To me it was an affirmation of so many things.

Oracle: Solomon's Seals, maybe that's an *anhangsel*.

Jack: It's the use of the Seals and more. An *anhangsel* does not necessarily mean just the use of a Solomon Seal from the sixth, seventh, eighth, or ninth Books of Moses. The protective value of the *anhangsel* is not dependent on the use of a particular seal. It's personalized in some manner. Some people use blood; some would use semen or menstrual blood if it were for a loved one. I always advise people to use their spit; after all, your entire DNA is contained in your spit.

Rose: Or a piece of hair!

Oracle: So what you're saying is, after you seal it up [the *anhangsel*], you need to personalize and charge it.

Jack: Exactly. It is an *anhangsel* from the moment it is personalized and activated. At that point, it has, to some extent, become alive.

Oracle: Like the ones of Christopher Whitt? [A famous 18th-century Hex-enmeister from Pennsylvania.]

Jack: Yep! I recently came across an article where they take a pendulum and use it with a circular board. This one they'd found was from the sixteenth century—found in the walls of an old German house, and the article stated that they weren't sure what it was used for. . . .

Oracle: I was told a story by Silver Ravenwolf about an old woman who had Alzheimer's, and yet when Silver burned her hand, the woman reached out and said, "Oh, you've burned yourself, let me fix that for you." She Powwowed for it and the burn went away. You blow three times with the same breath. . . . That's what I did for Michelle.

Rose: I did it for myself when I burned my hand on the stove.

Oracle: Why not? Hex is practical!

Rose: I try to make my water boil faster, but it just doesn't work! [*Laughter*]

Oracle: I've tried that, but it really takes some effort.

Jack: To do what?

Oracle: To make the water boil faster!

Jack: You can do this?

Rose: I'm trying!

Oracle: Me, too, but I can't; but Silver can, she just holds her hands out and. . . . [*makes bubbling sounds*].

Rose: I remember my grandmother cooking and chanting. I wish so much she was alive. I'd be like a sponge with her. When I was seventeen, I looked into Wicca, and my mother was so afraid of it, I promised her I was not going to touch it. That was the problem! She had the gift and was afraid of it. She could predict what people were going to have when pregnant. My girlfriend says to this day, "Your mother wished those boys on me!" [*Laughter*] My mother had it, but she didn't use it unless you crossed her. She wouldn't do anything outright but she'd say "I don't get mad, I get even." Sure enough, someway, somehow, she'd get even. She wouldn't chant, or do anything overt.

Jack: You don't have to. In higher levels of magic, you supposedly just think it and the chain of cause and effect begins. . . .

Rose: I can do that once in a while; I need to get worked up. . . .

Oracle: Me, too! Sometimes it freaks me out when it works.

Jack: Usually it is anger or rage. You need to say to yourself, "Stop before this gets out of me [as a projected thought]; don't send this out." To do a binding, is like that. You can bind people mentally, through projection. I learned that from an old black preacher. You just begin winding a band of light around the person, starting at the feet and circling around the head, till they're enveloped in the light of love, in the power of Christ's name. This way, they can't hurt anyone, and hopefully, the love will change their heart in some manner. You say, as you wind, "I commend (person's name) to the love of God, in the name of Jesus Christ."

Rose: It's not in front of this person?

Jack: Nope, just in your mind. You build a construct around them that protects you and does not hurt them. It works amazingly well.

Oracle: I know of a Hex who does something very similar. She just makes believe that she's wrapping them like a mummy. Especially if there is an abusive person or a criminal she wants to have caught. She says it usually isn't too long before they're caught.

We then moved to the subject of reading the signs and omens that are present in the natural world and give information about events to come.

Signs and Omens

Oracle: I remember when my mother's mother was dying in the hospital. I was living with my mother at the time. The night before she passed away, I felt like I just wanted to open the front door, and when I did, the wind blew in, and I could swear I could hear a lady crying. I'm not crazy, but I heard it, though I could not see anything. It was not a wailing but just a lady crying. That shook me up right away because I knew that kind of thing was possible from the legends, but you just don't think you'll ever really hear it.

Turns out that was the time my grandma's condition took a turn downward. I know I'm not crazy.

Jack: I know. I don't have any doubts. . . .

Rose: *[Whispering]* Oh, yes he is! *[Laughter]*

Jack: Well, then, we all are!

Oracle: *[to Rose]* I'm crazy about you!

Rose: Hah! *[Laughs]* I had had an earlier telephone conversation with Oracle centering on his personal vision for the future of Powwow.

Jack: One thing I'd like you to do for me. You have an interesting vision for the future of Powwow we've talked about this in the past. Tell me about it again.

Oracle: Well, you know Karl Herr and Lee Gandee and others have spoken of using Powwow in a Christian manner. Lee certainly was okay with that, but he knows that this stuff predates Christianity and doesn't always follow the traditional or official Christian line, no matter how much we may try to cover for it. Karl Herr says it's rooted in the Christian faith with elements of Kabbalah and other stuff. Powwow is a magical practice, which the church officially frowns upon even though their own holidays, liturgical elements and rituals like communion, and invocations are often magical in intent and are borrowed from earlier traditions. If you also look further you begin to recognize elements of indigenous Germanic practices such as the *Himmelsbrief*, the *anhangsel* and so forth. In this you are not dealing with Christianity or the Kabbalah but old German Heathenism. My vision is to be able to restore Powwow to a valid spiritual path that a person could walk if they so desired.

Jack: A spiritual path for a neopagan?

Oracle: Right! I want to restore Powwow to its ancient roots as much as possible with reference to the old Germanic pantheon and uncover, as completely as possible, its original shamanic practices. There are, I believe, a lot of people who want to walk the neopagan path but can't buy into the whole Wiccan thing. Some go into the Celtic

Reconstructionist path, the Strega, the Asatru and so on. The Gard-
nerians are making the claim that everything original came through
them, and they are the only true path to divinity. They call out to
a litany of Gods and Goddesses from all pantheons. The point is, in
magical traditions for Germans, it would have been German deities,
not a hodge-podge of divinities. In one of the famous German
witch trials, the woman talked of shamanically traveling to visit
Frau Holda in her cave and learn the future. We used Frau Holda
in that recent spell as well as the German God and Goddess of
justice. [Oracle was referring to an incident where the Hex community gathered to do a binding on a local rapist who had assaulted
Oracle's fifteen-year-old niece.]

Jack: Aren't you risking, with such an ethnic approach, a comparison with
some right-wing elements of the Asatru movement, or a comparison
with the quasi-occult, pseudo-religious practices of the Nazis?

Oracle: The point is that the Nazis, like all power-hungry groups, borrowed
and perverted the memories of their ancestral religion to serve their
own political and social ends. Most people do not remember, or try
to forget, that Hitler also went around Germany and received the
blessings of the various Christian denominations before going about
his dirty work. Seriously, I'm not out to serve any political or social
end but to restore, if I can, a valid spiritual path and make it available
to those who might be drawn to it. The Nazis were certainly not
the only group who have misused religion to their own political
ends. Just watch the news. Thank heavens, we have the separation
of church and state in this great country. The mix of religion and
politics has covered the world with blood many times over, no
matter whose God or Goddess was supposedly in charge. Thomas
Jefferson knew this, and that's why he wrote what he did.

Jack: Understood. So, what you would like to do is evolve Powwow. . . .

Oracle: Back to its original Germanic forms, before it started to take on
all these additional influences. Have you ever asked yourself why
it took on these influences? It did it to survive, to protect and
preserve itself in the face of and from persecution. As you know

from your study of the Inquisition, entire villages were persecuted, wiped out for the wrong beliefs, and nowhere was it more ruthless and thorough than in Germany.

Jack: I've read that there were villages in Germany where the entire female population was put to death. I read recently that if you were declared a witch, your property was seized and handed over to the church even after you were dead. There were caravans laden with personal effects and personal property moving across Europe to Rome in a constant stream during the four hundred years of the Inquisition. Much of the Roman church's wealth and land holdings came from this practice. Sort of makes you wonder about motivation, doesn't it!

Oracle: Exactly. It also puts a squelch on any future resistance. There is a book by Stephen Flowers that you must read—*Galdrabok: An Icelandic Grimoire.*

Jack: Lee seemed to think Powwow went back to India. What does this guy say?

Oracle: Well, he says here, "This healing spell corresponds to one in the Rig-Veda."

Jack: No kidding! He's found that connection, too!

Rose: *[Laughing]* You need to buy this book, don't you!

Oracle: German magic has taken on many regional forms and even differences between northern and southern practices. Flowers found this stuff in Icelandic grimoires and brought it forth as Teutonic magic. Look at this rune, a six-pointed star. What does it resemble?

Jack: A hex sign.

Oracle: Right! It a rune of the snowflake . . . used for protection and shamanic travel. It is the rune of Frau Holda. He [Flowers] also mentions Lee and *Strange Experience.*

Jack: I've got to find this book!

So ends the interview of January 2003. Oracle, Rose and I have kept in touch and they continue to grow as Powwows and people. We often get together on the telephone to discuss ideas and to help each other magically. Oracle is currently preparing a text of his own based on translations of traditional German grimoires.

There are many other stories concerning Powwow with which I have been involved that are not connected with Oracle and Rose but which illustrate the persistence of Powwow as a magical tradition. Here is a recent story.

"Can You Help Us, Sir?"

In April 2004, my wife and I went on a camping trip in Western Tennessee. After a cold winter, we both needed a chance to secure the peaceful presence that can be found so easily in attractive natural surroundings. We went to one of Tennessee's wonderful state parks, set up our tent, hiked and rested. As it was before the busy camping season, we and a few other campers had the place to ourselves. We tended to gather to chat under the large pavilions provided by the campground. We all shared our stories and our common interests. I mentioned that I was in the process of writing this book and briefly described the subject matter. I noticed a well-dressed family at the edge of the group who seemed to react intensely to my story. Given their conservative dress and demeanor, I assumed that I had trod upon someone's theological toes.

As we were all getting up to leave, that same couple came over and approached my wife and me. The man introduced himself and said, "Can you help us, sir?"

I noticed the serious tone and realized that this was not going to be an ordinary comment, so I replied, "How may I serve you?"

"Well, you see," he said, "my wife's ex-husband's family has placed a curse on us!"

"How does it show itself?" I asked, trying to get clues as to what was going on and maybe deduce if this was a real manifestation or the result of a bitter divorce proceeding.

He began to relay a series of accidents, unusual illnesses and strange events that had all the characteristics of a projected curse. I thought to myself, "This person has risked a great deal to reveal himself and his family to me this way, the least I can do is to treat him and his problem with respect."

I said to the distraught man, "I believe I can help you." I began to describe how to spiritually make one's home secure from spiritual attack by lining the windows and doorways with salt. I recommended bringing iron implements into the house, a floor wash of Van Van Oil and the sprinkling of powdered Angelica root. As I was currently making charms for friends who had requested them, I secured my box from the tent and made them a protective red mojo bag of a whole Angelica root, dressed with lodestone and High John Conqueror Oils, right there at the pavilion. I made the sign of the cross on the women's forehead with holy water and said a brief prayer on her behalf.

The couple thanked me profusely and returned to their rather impressive RV. Later that night, they offered my wife and me a glass of homemade wine as a gesture of thanks. Throughout our contact, they presented themselves as utterly sincere, decent, hard-working people, who had very traditional values and beliefs. After I returned home, I made another, more elaborate, charm and mailed it to the couple, who had given me their home address. I trust and pray they have found some relief and release from their troubles.

While I was assisting this family, I noticed another camper looking upon all of this with no small measure of astonishment. He later walked over to our tent and said, "If I had not seen that with my own eyes and ears, I would have never believed it! Those people were educated! How can they believe in spirits and curses in this day and age? With modern technology, the Internet, and everything, I thought this stuff was long gone."

"I'm afraid not," I replied, remembering the advice once given to me by Mr. McTeer (see Chapter Two: Interview: James E. McTeer, "The White Prince"). "There is a part of all of us, where lives, no matter how sophisticated or educated, a place where we hold to the possibility that something might just exist beyond what we can scientifically verify. This is the part of us that nurses the belief in life after death, that some Divine being, somewhere, is concerned with our personal well-being, that two thousand years ago, a Jewish holy man, condemned for sedition, crucified by the authorities, arose from his grave and lives eternally in a paradise somewhere, waiting for our appearance at his door. These folks were wise. They paid attention to their beliefs and sought what they knew and believed was an acceptable solution. To deny it would have pushed this belief back further into their minds, causing untold sorrow and trouble. In reality, theirs was a healthy response. It is as simple as that!"

"I see what you mean," he replied. "I just never would've believed it!"

"There are many worlds within this one, many realities, many states of being; you've just witnessed one more,"   I said.

He smiled and headed back to his campsite.

"That's what I like about you!" my wife remarked. "Life with you may sometimes have its moments, but it's never dull!"

I remembered and repeated Lee's words, "Life itself is the greatest magic of all!"

Due to the enhanced communications available on the Internet, people have found me and have sought spiritual counsel. While I often speak on various spiritual topics, I will not be a spiritual teacher to anyone, but I will respond to sincere seekers as best I can. The following exchange came about as a result of several workshops I conducted at an alternative spirituality retreat in western Tennessee in the Spring of 2007. Here's an excerpt from our online correspondence:

Dear —————,

I'm back in town and rested so; let me try to answer your questions.

Question 1:

My spirituality has always been life-permeating and intense, but casual. I have not practiced devotionally. In the couple of months prior to the festival, I was being led to look at beginning to incorporate devotional ritual as part of my day. I don't know where to begin . . . Would be grateful for any advice. My relationship with deity is personal and interior, conversations, energies, etc. I would like to work on how to bring more intent and purpose into my interaction with the Divine in a devotional way. The question isn't about the trappings of spirituality but about how to "work" ritual/devotion into a daily approach to Deity.

Answer:

I am really happy that you are considering incorporating devotional practices into your spiritual life. Many modern people shy away from private devotion but, I believe it to be at the heart of personal spiritual and psychic growth. First, I can only give you advice that has worked for me so, here goes:

I set aside sacred space for this practice. In the corner of my bedroom I have an altar discretely set up on top of a bookcase. I have various images that are spiritual focus points for me. I also personalize it with my wedding rings and devotional beads/malas.

I set aside time each day for a devotional practice. For me, I get up a bit earlier than Lesley, and go and stand at my altar. First I greet the images of the Divine that are pictured there. I offer my welcomes, prayers and praises and then just stop talking and thinking and listen. Listening is critical. Over the years this has become a normal part of my morning routine. It now takes only 5 to 10 minutes but does a world of good in how I end up approaching the day. In addition, the altar space itself has developed a presence of its own that I feel as I come into its presence. The same thing happens at sacred shrines. The physical space becomes "charged"—for lack of a better word.

When I come home at night I repeat the ritual before retiring to bed. Before leaving and when returning from a trip, I visit the altar and deities. Sometimes it is just a greeting or I say thanks for a safe trip. I've been doing this for 27 years in multiple locations and have gained invaluable benefit. I remember it seemed awkward at first, but I grew into the practice. I also conduct private meditations when I am troubled and need to talk to the Divine or just want to feel that Divine presence. You will find you grow to really enjoy it. The daily focus in the Divine in one's life can be an ongoing source of growth and life support. What you say or do is not critical but must be sincere. The Divine will not deny him/herself from you if you reach out with your heart. I promise you this. Just remember to listen.

Question 2:

From the "Spirits" class: I attended the class less out of interest in ghosts (although it was fun to hear people's stories) but more out of interest in learning how to open myself psychically (safely). I'm very spiritually sensitive and energetically sensitive, but there is a thin eggshell between me and "psychic" experiences . . . a deep unconscious fear that pushes me into the mental realm, analysis, etc. instead of staying with and feeling the experiences that come from the ocean of consciousness all around us, with all its layers. My question is—you alluded a couple times to there being ways to start practicing, training yourself to open and receive.

Answer:

Devotional practices are always a good beginning. Nature has always been a source of comfort and strength for me so, long walks in silence in a woodland area or even a park will work well. If you feel you must take someone along for safety, explain to them that this is for spiritual practice and you enjoy their presence but silence is critical. You will find that you begin to intensely listen to the sounds around you and as the "ever-talking mind" finally calms down, you will be unconsciously opening to the world that your mind normally shuts down or blocks. Feel the air on your skin and become aware of its presence as you go deeper into trance. You will also begin to sense the "mood" of energy of the area. If you feel impelled to stop walking, do so and find a quiet, comfortable space. Mentally surround yourself with protective energy, but do not close down your awareness. Remain absorbed in listening and open your consciousness. It may take awhile to get this practice down but when you do, you will know it.

With time, as you continue, you will start to hear and see that which is hidden. It will come in the form of little voices, little touches and maybe even visions.

Practice and cultivate your time of silence and solitude, taking care to slowly bring yourself back into regular awareness when you are ready. After a while, you will be able to open yourself at home or outside. You will pass people on the street and know what they are thinking and feel their energy. This will eventually translate into the ability to sense non-embodied life forms in everyday settings. Learn to turn your enhanced awareness on and off. This is essential and for your own safety. I always feel the presence of spirits or ghosts via touch. My body and especially my hands have, over the years learned to encounter and detect their presence. Learn to trust your perceptions and accept the validity of the encounters. They are happening. This is difficult for many folks because of the way we have been acculturated, but push through your rational mind's attempts to hold you in its grip.

Question 3:

From the "Cosmic Chaos" class: At one point you said something (and tried to repeat it) about the emotional level of moving energy. I wish I could remember what you said. I hoped for a chance to go back to it, but the class discussion was quickly taking on momentum of its own, and there was no way back to your point. It is what stood out to me in *The Secret* [referring to the recent book by Rhonda Byrne] as well—that there is an emotional connection, not just thoughts. You said something very simple about directing energy and pushing it and . . . something about emotion. Do you recall? Can you explain?

Answer:

All life, thought and awareness is energy in various degrees of density and intensity. Within the human mind, we use emotion to motivate and direct our mental energy. Emotion is the method or vehicle for concentrating our psychic energy and pushing it toward a thing we desire or wish to accomplish. It is the method by which a Powwow or other shaman heals. To project that energy I pull it into my heart chakra and mentally push it out through my arms and hands to a source. Here's a way to get used to pushing energy:

Find someone you trust and who agrees to work with you. Ground yourselves personally and then sit across from each other and extend your arms, palms facing each other. Put your palms together, feels each other's energy build up and then slowly start moving your palms back toward yourselves until the connection breaks. With practice, you will soon be able to send energy back and forth to each other. If you use emotion to focus and direct that energy, you will see dramatic results. Use love rather than anger to move your energy, for the safety of the other person. Even sexual energy can be employed in this manner but make sure the other person is okay with this.

May your life be filled with Divine joy, healing and blessings,

Jack

CHAPTER 10

The Appalachian Granny-Woman
The Magic and Wisdom of the Mountains

The ordinary acts we practice every day at home are of more importance to the soul than their simplicity might suggest.

—Thomas Moore, (1779-1852)

Formerly, when religion was strong and science weak, men mistook magic for medicine; now, when science is strong and religion weak, men mistake medicine for magic.

—Thomas Szasz, *The Second Sin*

WHEN WE HEAR the word Appalachian today, a variety of images comes to mind, ranging from the beautiful mountain vistas found in our national parks, to the traditional art and music that enjoys worldwide popularity, to the struggles and trials of its people to maintain their traditional way of life in a modern world. These mountainous areas, spanning thirteen states from Maine to Georgia, and reaching heights of over 4,000 feet, were once seen as a barrier to westward expansion.

Early colonists in South Carolina settled the lowlands and later, the Piedmont areas of the state. Only the hardy and desperate ventured into the mountains. The Native Americans, already under great social pressure and pushed out of their traditional lands, were no longer welcoming to those who encroached upon their final lofty sanctuary. Until 1763, when the Treaty of Paris ceded these lands to the English, the land beyond the mountains was the domain of the French, who were exploring and settling the Mississippi Valley.

Soon after the Cumberland Gap was discovered in 1750, people began moving through but not necessarily into the mountains, preferring the flat, fertile lands to the west. This period also coincided with the great displacement and subsequent diaspora of Celtic peoples from Ireland and Scotland. Following several failed attempts at independence, many Scots were forcibly removed from their traditional homelands, which were taken by the English government. The Irish potato famine forced hundreds of thousands to flee their ancestral homes for the great unknown of America. Many of these people, as we have seen in earlier chapters, were brought here under conditions akin to slavery: indentured servitude.

Moving down through the valleys of Pennsylvania and Virginia, the Scottish and Irish immigrants sought land but found little that was available and affordable in the settled areas. They also often encountered considerable bigotry from the people they met as they traveled southward. Many were scornfully labeled "Red Legs," "Hillbillies," and "Crackers," by some English settlers who were still prejudiced against their Celtic neighbors. The new immigrants sought somewhere to live free from such hostility. They wanted to build a society of their own, where they would be respected and welcomed and could recreate a form of the traditional society they once experienced. In South Carolina, the cultures of the Low Country and the Piedmont, or upstate, became distinct and slightly antagonistic toward each other. The Low Country folks saw their upland neighbors as dour, overly serious and lacking in education and culture. In his book entitled *Carolina Piedmont Country*, folklorist James Coggeshall illustrates the corresponding attitude of the up-country settler to their Low Country counterparts, when he recounts the famous upcountry joke:

In what ways are Charlestonians like the Chinese?

The answer: They both eat rice, worship their ancestors, and speak in a foreign language. (6)

Many of the settlers in the up-country also fled the cruel institution of indentured servitude and knew that if they made it into the hills, they would not be pursued by their "masters" or the professional bounty hunters sent to find them. Here, in the geographical isolation of the mountains, they were finally free to build their own destiny. Theirs would be a different world than the aristocratic planters of the coastal areas and the Piedmont farmers. Theirs was a world based on their memories of the Celtic values, laws and society of their homelands in the British Isles. It must be noted that while many other ethnic groups also moved into the Appalachians, including the French, Germans and African-Americans, they tended to assimilate into the dominant Irish and Scottish culture. Richard Maxwell Brown, in *South Carolina Regulators*, describes the situation in the colony as "fragmentary and divided. The four counties in upstate South Carolina were merely vague geographic entities possessing neither officials nor powers" (14).

Enterprising farmers hauled produce and trade goods to the Piedmont and Low Country, but the need for social and cultural reciprocation was not acknowledged or returned. Requests were made for such essential services as teachers, ministers and the like. Such requests were seldom heeded, as evidenced in the historical chapter on Powwow. As the population of African slaves surpassed that of the whites of the Low Country, the aristocratic culture began to see the need to create a human barrier against encroachment on their lands and status. The perceived threat was the possibility of slaves revolting or escaping into the frontier and possibly aligning themselves with the Native Americans. It was only then that the wealthy planter society of the Low Country began to cultivate positive relations with the citizens of the backcountry, who while not hostile, were understandably indifferent to the plight of the plantation owners.

It was also at this time that the planter society began to recruit and settle Germans into the Piedmont, as noted in the chapter on Powwow. Along with the establishment of a society somewhat disconnected from the planter society in the Low Country, there was the establishment of cultural medical traditions and practices. According to Anthony Cavender, in *Folk Medicine in Southern Appalachia*, "Ninety percent of the settlers of the southern Appalachia came from the 'British Borderlands,' an area encompassing northern Ireland (Ulster), lowland Scotland, and northern England, and of these groups the Scots-Irish were predominant" (31). These peoples had "a mixed ancestry representing in varying proportions Celtic, Roman, German (Anglo-Saxon), Viking, Norman and Gaelic origins" (Cavender 31).

The Magical Environment of the American Colonies

Most of the early English colonists, and later, Americans, believed in some element of the supernatural. They also brought with them to the new colonies a belief in the reality and presence of magic. With that belief was an awareness of those who could practice magic in some form for good or bad results. In almost every settlement, there were those who would be considered magical professionals. These were interchangeably referred to as charmers, cunning men or women, granny-women, power or moon doctors, witches, and wise-women, to give a few of their varied titles.

Few actual magical professionals made a living from their practice, although most folks performed small magical rituals designed to protect them and their properties from negative magic. Douglas Winiarski, in the *Encyclopedia of American Cultural and Intellectual History,* describes some regional practices:

> Cakes baked from flour and urine unmasked the identity of afflicting witches; horseshoes hung over the door, pins driven in to floor and witch-bottles buried beneath the hearth protected houses from the intrusion of supernatural agents. . . . In the Carolina backcountry moreover, spiritual vigilantes, known as witchmasters, peddled their countermagical services to families afflicted by neighborhood sorcerers. One such adept, a Revolutionary War veteran named Joshua Gordan, composed a book of spells designed to undo the damage caused by attack magic such as the "evil eye." (100)

In Appalachia, people also sought to retaliate against those they believed had attacked them using supernatural means. Michael Frome, in *Strangers in High Places: The Story of the Great Smokey Mountains,* recounts advice given him:

> If a certain old lady had bewitched a man or boy, he should draw a picture of that person with a representation of a heart upon it, then take the picture into the woods and fasten it to a tree by driving a knife through the heart. This action, coupled by refusing to lend anything to the "witch" would cause her to grow sick and lose her power. (247)

In 1997, an informant, who is a well-educated woman from Missouri and of Appalachian heritage, told me that on one occasion she witnessed her mother magically stop a certain neighbor from stealing milk. Her mother dug a hole in the barn where the family cow was kept, poured milk from the afflicted cow into the hole, and pounded the milk in the hole with a stick cut for that purpose, while chanting a certain incantation. Within a day, the neighbor appeared at their home, bruised, battered and begging forgiveness. She paid her mother for the milk, and promised never to do it again.

There was a common belief that a witch could steal milk from a cow at a distance by tying a dishrag to an axe handle and performing sympathetic magic. The witch accomplished this by milking the dishrag into his or her pail, while chanting a specific incantation. The cow may not have left the barn, but it would be unable to give milk when conventionally milked, which was a sign to the farmer of bewitchment.

Douglas Winiarski describes another common magical practice among conventionally religious churchgoers called bibliomancy: "Many pious Christians practiced bibliomancy, a divination technique in which one's future was predicted by opening the Bible randomly" (100). I have observed this form of divination practiced among urban and well-educated people. The idea is that, through supernatural intervention, the petitioner's attention will be drawn to a verse or section of the Bible that will provide a Divine answer to her or his question or insight to a problem.

In those early times, many people who were functionally literate kept written records of herbs, spoken charms and with formulas for material charms along what illnesses they cured. These practitioners of magical healing kept diaries or journals, just as many herbalists and witches do today. In colonial times, newspapers and broadsides posted on buildings and in public places proclaimed the benefits of homegrown cures and spells. Prayer groups were as common then as they are today. Church members concentrated on their repentance and their appeals to the Divine, hoping to secure spiritual relief from their suffering and that of their neighbors. Most modern Christians probably do not recognize the historically magical underpinnings of their actions. In fact, most churchgoers and clergy can find, in the Bible, the verses that provide scriptural legitimacy for those actions.

Many religious people have seen personal success, wealth and good health as favor and reward from the Divine. Conversely, throughout the 18th century, says Winiarski, "German pastors, for example, recorded hundreds of encounters with parishioners who ascribed their illness to human sin and pleaded for spiritual intervention" (101). Later, upon the belief that they had received a positive result from their efforts, parishioners would often commit themselves to the mission and work of the church as a gesture of gratitude. Winiarski also notes, "Protestant devotional behavior, in turn paralleled Roman Catholic practices in which lay-men and women sponsored feasts and masses to celebrate the healing intercession of patron saints" (100).

This was also a time when settlers and magical practitioners sought trance states, received visions and sought to interpret dreams. They were often skilled at reading omens regarding agriculture, childbirth, marriage and even the weather. Many of these omens have made their way into modern times. Marjorie Rowling, in *The Folklore of the Lake District*, attributes this familiar saying to the Scotland Lake District:

Red sky at night, shepherd's (or sailor's) delight,
Red sky at morning, shepherd's (or sailors) warning. (103)

People also believed in the protective powers of certain trees, such as the use of a forked wand from a hazel bush for discovering sources of ground-water (also called water-witching), which was also common in Appalachia and throughout the colonies. Rowling describes the process:

The straight handle of a forked branch is held in the right hand of the outstretched arm as the "dowser" walks over the ground to be tested. The folk twists and dips as it passes over hidden water, that is if the diviner himself possesses the necessary power. (97)

Another imported belief concerned the magical or protective power of certain naturally occurring items that could be worn as amulets or carried upon the person. An excellent example was the "Holed" or "holey Stone", a stone with a naturally formed hole in it. In Hertfordshire, England, flints with holes were employed for protection of the home. According to Doris Jones-Baker, in *The Folklore of Hertfordshire*, they were also used "to pre-vent horses from sweating by keeping away the dreaded 'night-hags' that got into the stables at night, took the horses and galloped them over the fields . . . before returning them, lathered with sweat, to their stalls" (95). In an interesting twist on such folklore, I was told that a holed stone, hung over the bedpost, would keep me from being "hag-ridden", a condition I regularly experienced before my sleep apnea was diagnosed and treated. I do, however, still keep a holed stone on the bedpost as a little bit of medicinal insurance, so to speak.

Aside from what may seem like irrational acts and ideas, one must remember that these were essentially pragmatic people and not given to flights of fancy or unnecessary actions. They believed in the effectiveness of their actions. During the same historical period in England, (1400–1600) many new urban dwellers professed skepticism, at least publicly, about the use of magic and other such metaphysical matters. Bob Trubshaw, in "Paganism in British Folk Customs," his critical analysis of the survival of pre-Christian elements in British folk customs, observed that even in the late-medieval period:

> Running in parallel were the ascending aristocratic interests in astrology and attempts to subdue 'witchcraft' and the various activities of 'cunning men and women. (par. 10)

The ambiguous characteristic of the cultural clash between the beliefs and sensibilities of urban and rural people continues to this day. It is not uncommon today to hear city-dwellers make fun of the manners and speech of their rural counterparts. Nevertheless, these urbanites may listen to traditional rural music on their stereos and iPods. Some things just don't appear to change with time. Outside the cities, however, just as in the British Isles, traditional beliefs still flourish as in times past.

Over the centuries there has been unconscious blending of the older religious concepts and practices into the popular religion of the day. Bob Trubshaw quotes historian James Obelkevich from his book, *Religion and Rural Society: South Lindsey, 1825–1875*, on these survivals:

> To use the term "paganism" for the non-Christian elements in popular religion [of the mid-nineteenth century] is convenient but misleading, since like popular religion as a whole, it was not a distinct and conscious movement or organisation but a loose agglomeration of religious phenomena. It was not a counter-religion to Christianity; rather, the two coexisted and complemented each other. (Obelkevich qtd. in Trubshaw, par. 23)

And concludes:

> It is hard to avoid the conclusion that paganism was dominant and Christianity recessive in popular religion. Paganism was rarely christianized, but Christianity was often paganized. (Obelkevich qtd. in Trubshaw, par. 24)

Magic was, like many spiritual practices, a response to an uncertain world. As Winiarski says in his section on the survival of such beliefs, "Godly Christians and religious visionaries perpetuated earlier supernatural beliefs as well" (104), and "Evangelicals and spiritualists, communitarians and medical sectarians, Indian doctors, slave conjurors all inherited a vibrant tradition of supernatural beliefs from the colonial period" (105).

Magical Inheritance from the British Isles

The tradition of the granny-woman in rural Appalachia is traceable in part to the village charmer, cunning men or wise-women, who has been part of rural life in the British Isles since ancient times. These shamanic healers, like their counterparts in other parts of the world, saw a two-level view of the causes of illness. Like many of their colonial neighbors, they believed that illness came from natural sources such as poisoned food, from injury or from an intrusion by some naturally occurring element, such as snakebite. There was also illness caused by the intrusion of a supernatural element into the person's life: a curse, invasion by an evil spirit or as punishment for some moral transgression or social taboo. Cavender says, "In the case of taboo, the sensate agent responsible for the illness was not a witch or sorcerer trying to cause harm, but the ignorant or neglectful sufferers themselves" (37).

To treat the illnesses resulting from natural sources or from personal ignorance or neglect, the role of the granny-woman developed in the mountains. Appalachian author Edain McCoy from *In a Graveyard at Midnight* notes that the granny-woman is considered an elder in the community and "in a region which has been long-noted for its distrust of modern medicine, it is often the granny women who are first consulted as to what cure to take" (11). Most granny-women read signs and omens associated with disease and illness and had a certain treatment for which they were known, such as the ability to "talk fire" (cure burns), stop bleeding or for curing certain childhood illnesses, such as whooping cough.

Transplanted Magical Therapies

Most Appalachians and other rural dwellers often employed incantations imported directly from the British Isles. Jacqueline Simpson, in *Folklore of Sussex*, includes this one, used for "Ague," or fever, which was self-administered:

> Ague, ague, I defy!
> Three days shiver, three days shake,
> Make me well, for Jesus sake! (103)

Many families also treated simple illness with a variety of methods and concepts regarding disease that date from the 19th century. Some are even traceable to ancient Greece. These responses or treatments usually consisted of attempting to restore the natural balance of certain fluids or "humours in the body," which they believed had been disturbed by contact with some disease-causing element. To treat these imbalances, they employed what is known as "heroic therapy," which involved, according to Anthony Cavender, "purging, bloodletting, sweating, blistering, puking and cupping" (39).

A remnant of these old medical skills is still practiced today in some Southern families. I can remember the time when having a fever meant being rubbed with a substance called Musterole, which smelled of camphor, and being placed under blankets to "sweat it out." In the early spring, we were also given a tonic by my grandmother, which usually included the laxative castor oil to purge any negative residues from our digestive tracts. Tobacco, moistened with saliva, was employed quite successfully to draw the venom out of insect stings. People consulted physicians but not as frequently as in today's society and only if home remedies proved ineffective. The uses of magically-based therapies were also employed when circumstance dictated and, according to Christina Hole in *Witchcraft in England*, "Since magic was essentially a neutral force, it could obviously be employed for good and evil purposes" (125).

Ginger Strivelli, in her online article "Appalachian Granny Magic," makes an interesting point regarding the word "witch" in the context of the granny-woman when she states,

> Amazingly, even the terms Witch, Witchcraft, spells, charms and such never became taboo in the modern Appalachian culture. Nearly every mountain top and "holler" community had their local "Witch" who was openly called such, as a title of honor, not as a insult or a charge of crime, as the term came to be used in other more urban American cultures of the seventeen, eighteen and nineteen hundreds. The "Witch Doctors" were still called upon to heal a sick child, or deliver a baby, or tend to the dying, as Witches had been so charged with doing in Europe during ancient times. Since often a mountain community had no medical doctor to call upon, the local "Witches" continued to work as the only healers, well up until the early twentieth century. . . . The local "Witch" was also called upon to dowse for water, ley lines, and energy vortexes when one was digging a well, planting a new garden, burying a loved one, or doing any other work with the Earth. (2).

The idea of an unnatural illness that resulted from a magical or supernatural intrusion was never acknowledged in my family as having any validity. The belief, however, in religious healings, miracles and to a lesser degree, the possible presence of spirits, was tolerated but not openly discussed. Nevertheless, for many other families such events were quite possible and considered normal, regardless of educational level and social position.

Black and White Magic

The type, intent and effect of the magic seemed to determine the overall social acceptance of such practice. Despite the often earnest assertions of the clergy and members of the professional medical establishment that it was all a matter of demonic origin or simple superstition, magic, as a practice, has persisted to this day. There was a clear distinction between black and white healing magic.

Black healing magic involved the reversing of a spell or curse back to its originator or the transferal of illness from the sick person to a thing or a creature. In Appalachia, I have heard of the act of transferring a fever into an uncooked egg or a raw potato as part of a healing ritual. The contaminated object is then buried in a neutral place; care is taken to not break the object, as doing so would release the illness back into the nearest person. In Appalachia, a red or black string was also employed to draw the illness into the string, which would then be destroyed by the healer, usually in a fire. A less humane version of this method involved transferring the disease to some unfortunate animal and then destroying it.

White healing magic, on the other hand, often involved the use of herbs and plants; the creation of charms to heal and protect the client; and the use of incantations and rituals, usually within a Christian religious ritual. One additional and very common form of white magical healing is known as the "laying of hands" on a person to draw out the illness or pain or to infuse the patient with healing energy from the healer. This method is still used by the witch, the granny-woman and the local preacher.

The Tradition of Charmers

In examining the cultural roots of the granny-women in Appalachia, it is critical to understand their counterparts in the British Isles. It is also important to note that most people in the rural areas of the British Isles were magically self-sufficient and viewed the practice of magic as a normal part of daily life. In rural England, notes Christina Hole,

> Most women knew a good many healing charms, some of them very ancient and rooted in pre-Christian paganism and many were versed in the making of love-charms, or the best way of calling home an errant lover. They also knew how to keep away evil during the night, to prevent horses from being hag-ridden, to protect the house from lightening and the newborn child from fairies and indeed, how to cope with almost every normal household peril or emergency. The farmer played his part in the magical observances that were absolutely essential at different seasons of the year. (126)

There appears to have been a distinction between the cunning folk and those called witches, although both types occasionally found themselves at odds with the law. Records and transcripts from 15th- and 16th-century trials in the British Isles, indicate the distinction was largely based on the type and amount of maleficent magic performed by the individual and from what supernatural source they drew their power. Both of these groups differed from the most common type of healer, the village charmer.

Owen Davies, in a 1998 *Folklore* article, "Charmers and Charming in England and Wales from the Eighteenth to the Twentieth Century," makes clear that "Charmers were quite a diverse group of healers" (41). Davies asserts that they have been often confused with the cunning man or white witch who practiced magic in a variety of ways that included spirit contact and interaction. Charmers were almost exclusively healers and, notes Davies, in the British Isles have "outlived most other aspects of folk magic, and charmers remained in demand in parts of the country up until the 1970s" ("Charmers" 41). Davies categorizes charmers into three groups based on their technique of healing: The first type of charmer used written or vocal charms, usually with an incantation; the second "had an innate healing touch" ("Charmers" 42) and the third used some object or charm to effect a healing. The charmers were distinct in that they only healed simple illnesses or wounds and were not considered to possess any other magical abilities. In all other aspects of their lives, they were just members of the community.

The charming tradition certainly made its way to America and remained strongest in rural and isolated communities. Nowhere was this more apparent than in Appalachia. Similar to their British ancestors across the sea, charmers would act upon request and were secretive about their methods or incantations. As in the Powwow tradition, such special knowledge was to be passed across gender lines and usually when death seemed near. I can remember giving a talk about folk healing in central Ohio a few years ago. After my talk a young woman named Sandy approached me and exclaimed, "I grew up in the mountains of West Virginia and my mother was a healer. She would speak over a burn and all the pain would go away. After your talk, I know why my mother wouldn't teach me what she knew! She told my brother and I thought she didn't trust or love me enough to tell me too. I've been angry at her all these years for nothing."

The Appalachian granny-woman was much more likely to be a charmer than a traditional cunning person. Certainly, the woman I will call Mrs. Sarah Ramsey, who was my main contact and of Scots-Irish descent, would fall more easily into the role of charmer, although she had other gifts and abilities. She also aided those who found themselves confronted by evil

influences and magical intrusions. The categories and distinctions often
applied to these people by scholars who study them are never as neat and
tidy in reality of daily life.

Also, like her British counterparts, the granny-woman tradition of Appalachia was not strictly a remnant of the culture of the British Isles. Like
the root doctor and the Powwow, they absorbed elements of magic and
practices from other groups, as well. These healers were too practical to
reject a technique that produced the required result simply because it came
from a group different from their own. Anthony Cavender says, "English
translations of German charm books, such as John George Hohman's Powwows, were consulted by Southern Appalachians" (45) and many practices
such as doing things in multiples of three and the use of certain colors for
magical charms were also borrowed from the Germans. Most people in the
back country did not concern themselves with the origins of the magic
they sought and employed. Historian Kay Moss, in her book, *Southern Folk
Medicine, 1750–1820,* notes,

> German Powwow Medicine traveled down the Great Wagon road during
> the mid-eighteenth century when the Shenandoah Valley of Virginia and
> the Carolina and Georgia piedmont regions were receiving the initial flood
> of European settlers. Notwithstanding, the name powwow remedies has
> no American Indian origin but stemmed from German practices. Gaelic
> knowledge of curative charms and incantations was equally rich. Sympa-
> thetic cures were introduced by Scots-Irish and other European settlers as
> well as Germans. With their own firm traditions of magical healing, many
> Euro-Americans readily accepted African conjuring. (153-154)

From the above-noted examples, and from any reflective study of the
folklore of magical healing, it is clear that these practices have been syncre-
tist: borrowing and synthesizing from many traditions and cultures over the
centuries. It seems pointless to debate or to try to pinpoint the minutiae of
the origins of such traditions, as so many are lost in the mists of time and
through the natural evolution of human culture and practices.

Cunning Folk: The Shaman of Rural Britain

If people in rural Britain had a problem beyond their abilities or that seemed to be of supernatural origin, they turned to the local cunning man or woman, who might also be called a white witch. Most cunning folk, like their neighbors, were engaged in the regular daily activities of an agrarian culture. They also engaged in typical shamanic activities such as healing; reading fortunes omens and giving oracles; divining the future; psychic discovery of missing persons, items or animals and even dowsing for new sources of clean, drinkable water. They cast spells for their clients. Some had a negative side to their practice. Like other shamans, they often were socially at the periphery of their communities, both sought after and scorned at the same time. All these activities occurred under the public condemnation of the church and civil authorities, who viewed such goings-on as backward superstition; however, the local shamans often were secretly consulted by those same authorities. Sadly, they also made easy scapegoats if some misfortune befell the population or region.

Some well-known cunning folk

Some cunning men and women actually became famous, including Tamsin, known as Tammy [Blight] Blee, from Cornwall, who began her career in 1830 and practiced throughout the 19th century. Researcher Jason Semmons says, on Owen Davies' Cunningfolk Gallery website,

> Many of Blight's customers were farmers who came to see her about sick cattle, others were young women anxious about their marriage prospects. In most cases Blight was able to provide uncanny cures that confirmed her magical reputation. ("Blight" par. 1)

Another famous 19th-century cunning man was Billy Brewer (1818–1890), who was known as the "Wizard of the West," (Davies, Cunningfolk Gallery, par. 2) and peddled his charms along with clay pipes door-to-door.

A 19th-century cunning woman with the odd name of "Daddy Witch," from Cambridgeshire, was as famous in death as in life. As it was commonly believed that she still followed the old pagan religion, when she died in 1860, she was refused burial in the church cemetery. Researcher Paul Grantham, in his online article "Daddy Witch's Grave: Horseheath. Cambridgeshire," says of this elderly woman:

When she died she was buried in the centre of the road leading between Horseheath and Horseheath Green, just where it passes a close opposite the sheep pond. (par. 1)

The grave was always identifiable by the bareness of the ground said to occur as a result of the heat which emanated from her body. Even during periods of heavy rain locals claimed that the area immediately above and around her grave remained dry. Local children were brought up in the belief that good luck would occur if they nodded nine times as they passed the grave. (par. 2)

A final notable cunning man was James "Cunning" Murrell (1780–1860) from Essex. Murrell was noted for his ability to heal animals, find lost items and reverse the spells of witches. Sue Kendrick, in her online article, "The Cunning Men of Essex," says:

He often referred to himself as the Devil's Master and claimed to be an adept at exorcising spirits, lifting curses and chastising witches. His witch bottles were well known and were used in conjunction with nail parings, blood, urine and hair. His success at dealing with witches who worked on the dark side was legendary. (par. 6)

Murrell was, like many cunning folk, known to be a flamboyant person, which enhanced his reputation. Kendrick says Murrell was

... the seventh son of a seventh son, which is said to confer the gift of second sight. A secretive man who traveled only by night, he was a skilled astrologer and herbalist and was often seen collecting plants by the light of the moon and suspending them from the rim of his umbrella. (par. 1)

Murrell, unlike many of his contemporaries, charged his clients for his services. Going to see Murrell was an experience in and of itself, as compiler George Knowles describes in his online biographical sketch, "James 'Cunning' Murrell (The Master of Witches)":

For his consulting room, Murrell used the front room of his cottage in which could be seen bunches of drying herbs hanging from the ceiling. In one corner of the room was a large chest in which he stored many of his magical textbooks and papers. In another corner a table on which could be seen a magical knife, a human skull and various other magical implements. Beneath the window was his desk and writing slope, with a high back chair in which he would sit and compile his notes and correspondences. To one side of the fire stood a large brass telescope and on the other side two more chairs for guests or patients. (par. 5)

Like Murrell, James McTeer and Lee Gandee realized the importance of establishing a magical/mysterious setting for their practice. To step into their domain was to enter a world apart and opened the client's mind to the experience they had sought by coming in the first place.

While cunning folk provided a range of magical services, usually each individual had a certain magical task in which they specialized, from finding lost relatives to speaking or making special charms or other protective implements, such as a "witch bottle." It is interesting to note that archaeologists and historians still find witch bottles and other magical charms and devices as they explore the old houses of America and the United Kingdom, which provide evidence of the enduring faith in magical activities. In his *Journal of the Royal College of Physicians—Edinburgh* article, "Illness without Doctors: Medieval Systems of Healthcare in Scotland," W. J. MacLennan says, "Despite advances made in orthodox medicine, many Scots continued to use folk medicines well into the twentieth century" (60). Such practices included the passing of sick individuals through the naturally occurring hole in a stone, "to cure sickly children or ensure an easy delivery" (MacLennan 60). He also describes the continuing practice of the sick visiting holy wells, which clearly dates from pre-Christian times: "After drinking the water, walked three times clockwise around it. When they departed they left an offering on an adjacent stone" (MacLennan 63).

In her book *In a Graveyard at Midnight,* Edain McCoy says that certain Appalachian cures involve waters that become imbued with healing powers, such as those collected on Ash Wednesday.

Most cunning folk were considered different than a village charmer or parish priest or vicar because of some extraordinary psychic or magical ability. This would often include the gift of prophecy and the ability to see accurately beyond the social masks people wear in daily life. Like her counterpart in the British Isles, McCoy says that the granny-woman, by virtue of her enhanced abilities, could function as a prophetess whose "predictions, traditionally given at Christmas and New Year's, are listened to carefully and heeded well" (12). The granny-woman was often believed to be able to deduce an infant's true character. She was often sought out to solve personal or family problems, much as a professional counselor is today. Also, like her British ancestor, she was the community historian in an often-illiterate culture. By virtue of her role as community counselor, she had access to knowledge that is generally kept from public view. This gave her a great deal of personal power, which could protect her or place her in peril, should she try to misuse it.

The Spirit Connection

In her excellent book, *Cunning Folk and Familiar Spirits: Shamanistic Visionary Traditions in Early Modern British Witchcraft and Magic*, scholar Emma Wilby traces the shamanic careers of both cunning folk and those considered witches. Wilby emphasizes the essential characteristic of the successful rural British shamans: a connection to the spirit world of helpful and harmful entities. The connection to these entities provided legitimization of the shaman's credentials, and a means of guidance as the cunning man or woman performed healings or other shamanic services. Like other shamans throughout the world, Wilby notes, "Cunning folk were also valued from their role as mediator between the living and the dead" (40), and today might often be classified as mediums or clairvoyants, particularly since the appearance of modern Spiritualism.

Meda Ryan, in her biography, *Biddy Early: The Wise-Woman of Clare,* describes this late 19th-century Irish woman as a "'Bean Fesa', Wise-woman or woman of knowledge" (101). Nancy Schmitz defines a Bean Fesa as "a type of go-between of the supernatural, the fairy world on the one-hand and the ecclesial world on the other" (qtd. in Ryan 101).

Throughout her life, Biddy Early, despite her remarkable record of successful healings, uncanny psychic predictions and personal generosity, was considered spiritually questionable by the local religious authorities. She had numerous negative encounters with local members of the Catholic clergy, who found her presence and activities theologically troubling and a threat to their status as spiritual leaders in the community. Mrs. Early never renounced her Christian faith but steadfastly maintained her right to pursue her magical life as well.

Local records indicate that at the time of her death and for decades afterward, Biddy Early was mourned by the community as a terrible loss. Ryan includes an excerpt from a local clergyman's eulogy of Mrs. Early, which reflects a modification of the clergy's former stance: "We thought we had a demon amongst us in poor Biddy Early, but we had a saint and we did not know it" (90). Ryan also noted, "twenty-seven priests attended her funeral" (90). Biddy Early was buried in an unmarked grave, as she never realized any real financial gain from her practice.

Mrs. Early's story was typical of the position in which many shamanic healers found themselves. On the one hand, respected and admired, on the other, distrusted and ridiculed, yet the tradition persists.

Shamans, spirit guides and gateways to the spirit world

Usually at some point in the shaman's life, a guiding spirit makes its presence known to a future cunning man or woman. This encounter with the world of spirits might later be recalled by the shaman as the impetus for choosing the life of a cunning man or woman, even if it was the result of accidental contact between the individual and a spirit entity. In the majority of cases, Wilby notes, "For both cunning folk and witches, the encounter with the familiar spirit was a visual one. They saw the spirit" (61).

A spirit might appear in a variety of forms from fairies to animals, as ghosts of relatives or as very attractive people of the opposite or the same sex. The style and nature of the relationship between shaman and spirit was decidedly and uniformly intimate, and often the cunning folk's familiars were often "given down-to-earth and frequently affectionate nicknames" (Wilby 63). While in a trance state, most modern mediums have one or more spirit guides who report to them.

As we will see in later chapters, the granny-woman I interviewed, "Mrs. Ramsey," did not appear to have a spirit companion. Nevertheless, I cannot help but reflect on Lee Grandee's relationship with his "boys." This super-natural, yet intimate, friendship was essential to Lee in accomplishing tasks such as retrieving hidden information or locating missing people or things.

An interesting modern historical case is that of Helen Duncan, a Scottish housewife and Spiritualist medium, who was accused of witchcraft and prosecuted during World War II. As of this writing, Mrs. Duncan's family is still seeking a full-pardon for her, which has been repeatedly denied. Apparently, during a séance, Mrs. Duncan communicated with the spirit of a sailor from a sunken British ship, which the government denied had been sunk. When this communication and its subsequent verification as fact became public knowledge, Mrs. Duncan was arrested and jailed as a spy and then a witch. Even after her prediction was found to be correct, she was held as a witch and jailed for nine months. Every legal effort was made to discredit her, without success. It seems the British authorities were concerned that she might accurately discern and somehow disclose the date of the D-Day Normandy landings. Mrs. Duncan's release from jail was not the end of her persecution by the authorities. In 1956, during a séance, while in a state of deep trance, she was forcibly manhandled by police and dragged away to jail. Her family asserts that the physical shock of this rough treatment of an elderly, frail woman led to her death a few days later.

Despite the world's current political problems, it is still difficulty for many of us to fathom what perceived threat could have led the authorities to behave in such a manner toward one of its elderly citizens. Even today, there are those in power who are apparently still threatened by others they view as having extraordinary abilities.

Spirit guides were also essential to lead and protect the shaman who traveled to the spirit world (often referred to as fairyland). The shaman would travel to the spirit world to receive training or to attend special events hosted by spirit entities. One interesting feature of this journeying was the real-world place where it allegedly originated. Most often a cunning person would claim to access the land of spirit from a locally known place deemed special, sacred or long associated with the world of spirits, such as an ancient burial mound, special cave, tree or spring. Biddy Early, the above-mentioned wise-woman of Country Clare, learned her healing arts from the fairies she consulted and was said to have visited a local fairy mound or Neolithic gravesite.

This concept of sacred or supernatural space appears to have migrated to the New World and to modern times. I remember a friend in college telling me of the ruins of a "little village" on some rural property owned by her parents southwest of Columbia, South Carolina. These little cottages were the size of a child's playhouse and had, in the 1920s, been the dwellings of a group of dwarves who lived in a retirement commune. The original occupants had either died or moved away, and the village was abandoned and in ruins. These ruins were thought by the community to be haunted or the source of some unearthly power. As my friend and I talked about this unusual place, she related a story. One afternoon, she and her high school friends had ventured into the village to explore it. She described feeling as if she had entered a dream world. She and her friends became disoriented and frightened, with one girl claiming that she could hear angry voices telling them to leave, which they did with great haste. I asked her if she could take me there sometime, and she adamantly refused, saying she would never set foot there again. Because of this frightening encounter, her father and his associates had destroyed the remaining buildings, and there was nothing left to see. Truly, for this modern, educated individual, this space remained a point of contact with some supernatural power.

Edain McCoy describes the Appalachian tradition of a praying-rock, which consists of a large stone or stone outcropping where prayers are offered and which people otherwise avoid. McCoy adds, "Around the praying rock are a collection of smaller stones, each one representing a person and need which is being worked on by the witch or preacher" (170).

The Role of the Granny-Woman as Midwife

In Appalachia and in rural Britain, giving birth and the delivery of a healthy baby were viewed as almost magical acts. In the days before hospitals and delivery rooms, birth was almost exclusively the province of women, with the granny-woman being the acknowledged expert. Most women in rural societies learned to deliver babies by assisting older women in the birth process. Males were usually banned from the actual birthing chamber. This was a woman's domain. A granny-woman would be called, and she would often stay in the home immediately preceding the birth and for a period of time after the birth, especially when the new mother had no other women to care for her and her family. Often other women friends or relatives would be present to assist the mother in preparing for the baby's arrival and making the items necessary for the baby's health and survival. One such item was a cloth strip called a "bellyband," used to protect the baby against umbilical hernias. This entire social system migrated from the British Isles and reestablished itself where great distance, poverty and lack of qualified medical practitioners were commonplace.

McCoy describes certain acts of sympathetic magic employed by a granny-woman to help ease labor pains, including placing a white stone or other sharp implement under the bed or mattress "to magically chop the pain into manageable pieces" (158). After the birth, the granny-woman examines the scene to see if there are signs or omens to be read. She will examine the umbilical cord of a woman's first child to determine the child's general health and "the total number of pregnancies the mother will have in a lifetime" (McCoy 158). As she examines and cares for the newborn, she is believed to be able to discern its essential character and much about its future.

Modern American society, upon rediscovering the people of Appalachia beginning in the 1920s, has not, until very recent times, treated its people, traditions and culture with the respect it deserves. A prime example of this is the manner in which the role of the granny-woman was treated by the medical practitioners, religious missionaries and social workers who spread out over Appalachia to bring the benefits of modern society to people they viewed as isolated and socially backward. According to Michael Frome in *Strangers in High Places: The Story of the Great Smokey Mountains,* the medical establishment took a very dim view of those "who administered herbs and potions with righteousness and ritualism" (248). Many granny-women, regardless of their record of successful healings and child-births, were derided as charlatans, causing many to be marginalized. Some were threatened with legal action and prison if they did not cease their activities. In the article, "Midwifery Work Came from Necessity," Lillye Younger recounts the story of a granny-woman from Henderson County, Tennessee, named Sallie Young and notes,

> Despite the fact that doctors frown on home delivered babies, Mrs. Sallie
> Young of Perryville bats 100 percent in her service as Midwife or "Granny
> women" as they were called. She never lost one. (1)

In summation, it is well to remember that the geographical and cultural isolation the Appalachian settlers experienced fostered a strong ethic of self-reliance and interdependence on one's neighbors when need or trouble arose. Like their pioneer ancestors, the communities of Appalachia were close-knit and often bonded by kinship and marriage. Once, while interviewing an informant in Camden, South Carolina, I was shocked to learn that during the Great Depression of the 1930s, the community had only one sheriff and one doctor for an area encompassing over 150 square miles, much of that only accessible by horse or on foot. Disputes and social problems were handled internally by the community. This casual form of law enforcement was common in Appalachia and in many areas of rural America long into the 1930s.

My late father, who was of Scots-Irish heritage, often relayed stories of the informal committee of men in the community who would act as the force of law, taking matters such as public drunkenness, adultery and other social infractions into their own hands. For example, if a man was discovered cheating on his wife, he was first given a verbal warning. If that was ineffective, other, more violent forms of persuasion were employed to restore social order or remove that individual from the community, one way or another. While this method of social control may have occasionally led to injustice or excess, one can imagine what might happen should these social conditions recur in our society due to natural disaster or political calamity. People in such communities and in the mountains never locked their doors, nor feared for their personal safety within the community. Their children were watched over by the entire community. This fierce personal independence and self-reliance, and the interconnectedness within communities helped to perpetuate the older tradition of the cunning man or wise-woman to the present day.

Rather than continuing with our discussion of Appalachian history and magical culture, let us proceed to my encounters with someone I call Sarah Ramsey, a true Appalachian granny-woman.

CHAPTER ELEVEN

Interview
Meeting the Granny-Woman

With age comes the inner, the higher life. Who would be forever young, to dwell always in externals?
　　—Elizabeth Cady Stanton, (1815–1902), *O Magazine,* October 2003

Angels and spirits are all around us all the time. You just have to be able to see them for what they are.
　　—"Sarah Ramsey," Virginia granny-woman

I BEGAN MY RELATIONSHIP with the granny-woman I will call "Sarah Ramsey" by hearing of her through her granddaughter, whom I will call "Mary." Mary worked with me as a student employee in the dining services at the University of Virginia in 1978–1979. As I was talking with her about my experiences with Lee Gandee during our work shift, Mary exclaimed, "My Grandma is a healer! She's healed everyone and helped deliver babies for years. You should meet her if you're interested in this stuff."

"I'd like to," I replied, "but I don't have a car."

"Well, call Momma [Helen Mayview] and ask if it's okay. Then if you want to go with me when I go visit, we'll ride together."

"Okay, I'll do that," I said. I was anticipating the chance to speak with Mrs. Ramsey about her healing practices. The next day, I dialed the phone number Mary had given me.

"Good morning. May I speak to Mrs. Ramsey?"

"This is her daughter, Helen Mayview. May I ask what this is about?" a voice answered.

"My name is Jack Montgomery. I'm a graduate student in Religious Studies at the University of Virginia. I was given your mother's name by your daughter, Mary, who said your mother was well known in these parts as a healer, and that she had helped people in this community for many years. I was wondering if I could come out with Mary and visit your mother. I also wonder if she would be willing to talk to me about her practice."

"My mother is getting on in years and doesn't do much of that sort of thing anymore. If she were to talk to you, what are you going to do with what she tells you?" Helen Mayview asked, clearly cautious about my intentions.

"I wrote my undergraduate thesis on healers, and I'm just interested," I replied.

"My mother doesn't have any formal education. What she does is a gift of God, and I don't want my mother put under the microscope or made fun of in some college somewhere."

"I assure you, Mrs. Mayview, with all my heart, that I have the highest respect for your mother's gift and will treat whatever she says with the utmost respect as the sacred gift that it is," I responded. "I also believe healing is the Lord's gift and do healings myself through the will and power of the Lord," I added, thinking I might as well insert this element into the dialogue to get through this barrier.

"Well, I suppose it would be all right then," Helen Mayview replied. "How about next Saturday morning, say round ten a.m.? You and Mary come on down to the house. Momma gets her hair done first thing Saturday morning, and we'll be back by then."

"That would be fine, Mrs. Mayview. Can I bring your mother a little something as a gift, something she likes?"

"That's not necessary," she responded, hesitated a moment, then added, "but we do like those Whitman's Sampler chocolates."

Whitman's Sampler it is." I smiled as I wrote down the request in my notes.

After I got this permission to visit with Mrs. Ramsey, I went on four separate occasions, with my friend Mary, to meet a truly unique individual.

That very next Saturday, armed with a large box of Whitman's chocolates, notepad and pens, Mary and I drove the roughly 25 miles through a series of winding rural routes, arriving at a small, modest, white farmhouse at the end of a long driveway. It was quite sunny and humid, and I thought to myself as I approached the front porch that I hoped they had a way to keep the candy cool. Soon the door opened to reveal a lady in late middle age, with her graying hair kept long in the style common in rural areas of Virginia. After she hugged her daughter Mary, Helen Mayview turned to me and said "You must be Mr. Montgomery, please come in and sit down; Mama will be out in just a minute."

"I hope this is the kind of candy you like," I said as I handed the box to her.

"Oh, this will be just fine, but you really shouldn't have." She smiled with obvious delight. "I'll just take this to the kitchen." Then she called toward the back of the house, "Mama! Mary and that young man from Charlottesville are here to see you!"

In a few moments, a small, thin, white-haired lady with piercing blue eyes came through the back hallway, wearing an ivory housedress and black orthopedic shoes. After she greeted her granddaughter, I rose and introduced myself, telling her how nice it was to finally meet her.

"I'm Sarah Ramsey," she said. "I'm seventy-seven years old, but I keep my own house and take care of myself. My daughter looks in on me and my son-in-law does my yard work now."

It was clear to me that she was establishing her independence. I thought how strong and dignified she looked, with her wrinkled hands reflecting a life of work rather than leisure.

"My husband Raymond has been dead for nigh-on twelve years. He was a carpenter by trade and kept a herd of beef cattle. He built most of these new houses in this area before he took sick," Mrs. Ramsey added.

As we talked for about 30 minutes, Sarah Ramsey revealed a life of initial isolation, economic frugality and a life lived by the seasons and close to the land. She wanted to know where I was from, who my parents were and how I came to be in Virginia. I finally opened the main topic of our dialogue by asking, "Ms. Ramsey, how did you come to be a healer?"

"Let's go outside where it's cooler, and we'll sit under the tree," she replied. "Helen, bring us a glass of that sweet tea."

Soon we were seated in folding chairs under a large oak tree. "My father—your grandfather," she said, looking over at Mrs. Mayview, "had the gift of healing. He could heal both man and animal; I suppose I learned it from him. He was a good Christian man and what he did came from God. That's why he never took money for it. We would be rich if he had, but he would have lost the power. People would come from miles around, sometimes in the middle of the night, and he would get up out of his bed and go to see about their sick child or horse. We didn't have any doctors nearby, and people had to look to themselves for help when they were sick. Nowadays, everyone goes to the hospital, but not back then—you couldn't afford it and people didn't trust hospitals and doctors."

"Did he teach you himself?" I asked, trying to draw out how the information and the tradition were passed along.

"As he got older, I suppose he needed someone to help him, and as I was the youngest [of six children] he took me along. I would watch as he drew the fire out of a bad burn or stop the blood, and I learned from watching and listening to him."

"What did you think of what your father's work?" I said, trying to discern how Sarah Ramsey herself viewed the practice at that time in her life.

"I knew it was God's work and that the Lord gave us the means to help ourselves!" she responded. "It is all in the Bible."

"How do you mean?" I asked. "Do you use a particular Bible verse?"

"Of course!" she responded. "It is in Ezekiel, where is says how to stop the blood!"

I learned later that she was referring to Ezekiel 16:6, which says:

And when I passed by thee, and saw thee polluted in thine own blood, I said unto thee [when thou wast] in thy blood. Live; yea, I said unto thee [when thou wast] in thy blood, Live.

I also learned that this particular verse was also widely used throughout the Carolinas for this purpose, along with certain passages previously mentioned (See Appendix). To perform the ritual, one whispers the verse over the afflicted area and the bleeding soon subsides.

"You mentioned that your father treated animals, Ms. Ramsey. Will the verse work for them as well?" I asked.

"Of course!" Sarah Ramsey responded, with a slight hint of annoyance. "We are all God's creatures, why shouldn't it work for them as well?"

"I mean no disrespect, I assure you!" I quickly responded, fearing she thought I was challenging her. "It's just that some people feel that you must believe in a healing for it to work."

"How can a cow believe? How can a horse believe? People can think what they will, it makes no difference. Son, this is the power of the Almighty moving through you—you don't even have to believe for it to work. If the Lord chooses you as his, it will work!" she replied emphatically.

"I believe you, Ms. Ramsey," I said, thinking I'd better change the subject, but Sarah Ramsey was not finished.

"I have seen my father stretch his hands over a horse they had given up for dead and pray, and by morning, the horse was up and around. This is by the will of God alone, and if the Lord wills you to heal, you will get better—no matter what the doctors say—but if he wills you to come home, [to die] nothing in this world can save you. A person with the gift is just an instrument in the hands of the Lord! That's the reason my father never took a dime for the healing he did for folks!"

"Mama, he believes you!" Helen Mayview interrupted at this point.

I was glad for the support and sought to turn the conversation to a more positive tone, in the interest of future conversations.

"Ms. Ramsey, when did you realize that the Lord had blessed you with the gift? Was it when you were helping your father?" I asked.

"No," Sarah responded. "I was headstrong at first, but then one day my brother was working on his old car and burned himself pretty bad. His hand was all blistered, and he was moaning in pain. Daddy was away on business, and Momma was at the neighbors. I was so scared, I finally went over and told him I would try to help him if he would let me. He said anything would be better than what he had, so I took his burned hand in mine and whispered the words as I sucked the burn out. Within an hour, the blisters were gone and so was the pain. Roy [her brother] said to me, 'Sis, I believe you got the gift!' I suppose I did, 'cause I been doing it ever since."

"Most people blow on a burn," I responded. "Why would you suck the burn out?"

"Because," she said, "blowing on a burn just drives it in deeper, like pouring cold water over it. You must suck the burn out like this!" She pursed her lips and inhaled sharply. "Then you blow the fire out to the side, like this!" At this point, she held up her hand, sucked the air from the back of her hand, then swiftly turned her head to the side and exhaled. She sank back into her chair, visibly fatigued.

"Momma, maybe we'd better go in now and rest." Helen Mayview spoke softly to her mother. "Mr. Montgomery can come visit us again sometime."

"I'd like to come back, if you think it's okay?" I said, hoping that I had not said or done anything to put her off.

"All right, son," Sarah Ramsey said, as she rose to go indoors. "Come back and we'll talk another time. It was nice to meet you." She moved with slow dignity off to the house on her daughter's arm, as Helen turned and smiled at me, waving good-bye.

Mrs. Ramsey's Magical Heritage

Two weeks later, we were again sitting under the massive oak tree in uncomfortable lawn chairs, as a pleasant breeze blew out of a deep blue, cloudless Virginia sky.

"Ms. Ramsey," I began, "you mentioned that you learned your healing from your father. Do you know how he learned it?"

Sarah Ramsey replied, "He learned it from his mother, my grandmother; she was also known for healing and for birthing babies."

"Oh, so she was a midwife?" I queried. "My great grandmother was a midwife in Camden, South Carolina. They said she delivered almost every baby in that area of town for about thirty years."

"My grandmother did the same!" Sarah responded. "I've delivered my share as well. Women back then didn't have any hospitals like nowadays, and not everyone knew how to do it, so they'd come or send for me, sometimes in the middle of the night, rain or shine, even in the snow. My husband would go to the door and then come back saying, 'Get up, so-and-so's having their baby.' I never refused to go, no matter what. Women had to look after themselves, especially when it came to babies."

"I remember Momma going out in the night!" her daughter Helen added. "Sometimes she'd come home crying because they'd lost the baby or the mother or both."

"They used to have 'childbed fever.' Sometimes there was nothing you could do for the poor little thing. It just wasn't meant to be." Sarah Ramsey seemed to drift away in reflection. I learned later that childbed fever was a term used to refer to various infections that could afflict the mother as a result of improper household hygiene or from a staph infection.

"How did you learn to do deliver babies? Surely your father did not do this sort of thing!" I asked, after a brief silence.

"Oh, Lord, no!" Sarah exclaimed. "I learned from my grandmother and my mother! I told you—womenfolk had to look after each other. No man was allowed near when babies was being born!"

It seemed to me that this seclusion or exclusion of the opposite sex had a practical side and was based in ideas of modesty, yet also had the component of a sacred gender-specific ritual. Here was a place and time when women were answerable mostly to themselves, as they conducted this most intimate of life's passages. I learned later that it was also women who presided over the preparation of a body at the end of life—especially a female body being readied for burial. Here again, men were excluded from this very private, sacred duty that the women performed for one other. These moments of transition were their private domain, their sacred space, their sacred ritual and duty. I learned that Mrs. Ramsey herself had lost a baby during the birth-process.

"It was stillborn—never had a chance," she quietly remarked, as she relayed this all-too-personal story of loss. "I told them to lay it aside in its crib. I got up the next day and washed and dressed it for its burial." She turned to her daughter, Helen. "Your father built its little coffin with his own two hands. Your brothers dug its grave."

The weight of her words told me she still deeply felt the loss and both her daughter and I were soon wiping tears from our eyes.

"Look at you two!" Sarah exclaimed. "Let's talk about something else!"

We sat for a while in silence; I was unable to formulate a comment or question.

"Show Mr. Montgomery how you 'call the birds,'" Mary, Sarah's granddaughter remarked finally. "I'll bet he's never seen anything like that before."

"I've always loved the birds," Sarah began. "My mother used to say that spirits and angels visited us as birds. One day, when I was by myself, I decided I would try to talk to them, and I found that I could."

Before I could formulate a response, being caught completely off-guard by this line of conversation, Sarah stretched out her arms and extended the first two fingers of her right hand.

"Come on," Sarah said quietly. "Come on, no one's going to hurt you."

As I watched, a small wren flew down form the oak tree and lit upon her finger. "Hello, pretty thing!" she said, as she lifted the little bird to her mouth and gently kissed its beak. She continued to talk to it in a gentle manner, much the way you would speak to a small child. The bird remained fixed upon her finger, turning its head from side to side until she said, and "Go on now, time to go!" At that, it flew away and disappeared behind the house.

"That's amazing!" I exclaimed. "Is it always that little bird?"

Oh, no!" she laughed. "Sometimes it's robins or even bluejays. I just know they're there and call them and they come."

"How do you know?" I asked. "Do you see them in the tree?"

"No." She smiled. "I know it in here," she said, pointing to her heart. "They know I won't hurt them, so they come to visit. I can't explain it to you. It just happens."

"She's been doing it as long as I've known her!" her daughter, Helen, added. "Birds have always been special in this house. Momma wouldn't let my brothers shoot anything that flies. Woe be to them if they did."

"The Bible says," Sarah interrupted, "'In as much as you have done unto the least of these; you have done it unto me.'" She added, "To hunt for food is one thing, to hunt for sport is a sin. That's what I believe!" Sarah sat back with a look of deep reserve and conviction. "God's creatures know who means them harm and who doesn't."

"They surely seem to know that you're their friend," I said, thinking of the legends that surrounded St. Francis of Assisi and his alleged ability to communicate with animals. Certain Hindu sages and Buddhist monks have also been said to possess such abilities, but I never expected to find such a person in the mountains of rural Virginia. "You mentioned earlier that your mother believed that spirits and angels appeared as birds? Could you explain that? How do you know?"

"The Good Lord has always had ways of sending us messages. In the Bible, they appeared to Abraham as people, so why not birds? Angels and spirits are all around us all the time. You just have to be able to see them for what they are," Sarah replied.

"But how do you know a regular bird from an angel or a spirit?" I asked.

"You know it in here!" Sarah Ramsey replied, pointing again to her heart.

Author's Note: It is interesting to note that author and historian Miranda Aldhouse-Green, in her book with Stephen Aldhouse-Green, *The Quest of the Shaman: Shape-shifters, Sorcerers and Spirit-healers,* traces the idea of birds and their connection to the spirit-world back to the mythological belief systems of Iron age Britain.

CHAPTER TWELVE

The Witch's Ball

Wisdom is not finally tested in the schools, Wisdom cannot be pass'd from one having it to another not having it, Wisdom is of the soul, is not susceptible of proof, is its own proof.

—Walt Whitman, (1819–1892)

. . . my Jesus is everywhere. No matter what happens, He is with me. He's loved me and has blessed me through all my troubles. Now I look forward to going home to be with Him one day soon.

—Mrs. "Sarah Ramsey," Granny-woman

IT WAS A CRISP AUTUMN DAY in November as I found myself seated in Mrs. Ramsey's living room. Her kerosene heater was attempting to take the chill away, and its faint odor filled the air. Mrs. Ramsey and her daughter, Helen Mayview, and her granddaughter, Mary Mayview, were also present. Mrs. Mayview made a sweet potato pie and coffee for my visit. After some small talk, I opened a subject I hoped would not upset her.

(*Author's Note:* Most of the following is dialogue, but there are occasional breaks in the interviews to include brief incidental information.)

JM: Mrs. Ramsey, I've been wanting to ask you about something since we first met. In all your years of helping people, have you ever encountered the practice of witchcraft?

HM: Mama, tell him about the witch's ball!

SR: No, it's best we not talk about such things.

JM: I'm very sorry. Please forgive me for asking.

HM: Mama, Jack's okay, go on and tell him. He may need to know what to do about it someday.

SR: *[after a long silence]* All right, Helen, help me if I forget.

HM: This all happened about ten years ago. Mama and I were sitting, watching TV and shelling peas, when we saw it rolling down the hall.

JM: What did you see?

SR: It was a witch's ball—a wicked spell that had gotten in the house. It was sent there to hurt us, to hurt me.

JM: What did it look like?

HM: Like a ball of hair with splinters and needles in it. It moved by itself.

JM: Were the windows open?

HM: No, it was so hot we had turned on the air conditioner. Anyhow, it turned and came into the kitchen.

SR: I knew what it was, 'cause I heard of them before. It's a thing with a will of its own.

JM: What do you mean? Was it alive?

SR: Sort of. A person creates it with their mind, gives it life and sends it out. If you don't see it and catch it, it will hide in your house and cause you no end of trouble.

HM: It came in the kitchen. I did not know what it was, so I screamed and jumped up on the counter. I spilt my peas everywhere. Mama just sat there and stared at it, then she pointed her finger at it and said something.

JM: Do you remember what you said, Mrs. Ramsey?

SR: I said, "Unclean thing, in the name of Jesus, I command you to stop! The Devil's work has no power here!"

JM: What happened then?

HM: It just froze! Then Mama got up and took an old Mason jar, put some Morton's salt in it and scooped it into the jar with the lid, all the while praying or something.

SR: I was saying the 23rd Psalm! "The Lord is my Shepherd. . . ."

JM: For protection?

SR: Yes.

HM: Then she screwed the lid on tight and carried it out of the house.

SR: I went and got a shovel and carried it to the woods and buried it under an oak tree. It's still up there now.

JM: How did you know what to do?

SR: I learned it from my mother's sister. She'd had a lot of trouble with some bad people who lived near her farm. They were fighting over access to the creek water, and they had sent several of these things after her. I don't know where she learned it.

JM: What would the salt do?

SR: It would break the spell. Like when a power line breaks and the electricity goes out.

JM: You mean it breaks the connection between the witch and the ball?

SR: Uh-huh! You see, there is a person that has made and sent the ball. They are in contact with it.

JM: Would the salt hurt them, too?

SR: It might give them a bit of a surprise! *[Laughs]* I've heard it burns them, like sticking your finger in a light socket.

This story reminded me of the mental energy projections used in Pow-wow and Hoodoo.

JM: I think I know what you mean. I used to know someone who could send out energy to heal people.

SR: That's what it should be used for! But you know, some people will always take what God has given us and use it for evil.

JM: I have to ask. Who do you think sent it?

MM: Oh, we know who sent it!

SR: Oh, I know who it was. My oldest son was dating a girl from a bad family. We could all see it, but you know how men get sometimes when a pretty woman looks twice at them. I'm sorry, I don't mean you.

JM: That's no problem. I know what you mean.

SR: Anyway, he finally came to his senses and broke it off with her. She blamed me for talking against her to him and went around telling people that she was going to get me. That just shows what kind of girl she was. I guess her and her mama got together and did it [the spell]. Her mama was known for doing that sort of thing in the past.

JM: Did you send a curse back to her?

MM: You should have!

SR: I most assuredly did not! I'm a better woman than that! The Lord said, "Judge not, that you be not judged!" I did my best to forgive them both and just moved on.

JM: Did you ever see another witch's ball?

SR: No.

At this point, I thought it best to drop this subject. The conversation then turned to more mundane topics until after lunch, when I ventured once again into uncertain waters.

JM: Mrs. Ramsey, I hope you don't mind me asking you, but have you ever seen a spirit or ghost?

Mrs. Ramsey just sat there, staring at the floor for what seemed an eternity. She always seemed to be weighing whether or not to answer me on these delicate topics.

SR: Son, I see them all the time . . . just like I see you and Mary and Helen. They are just not as solid.

JM: Can you talk with them? Do they try to tell you things?

SR: Yes, just like we are talking.

JM: What do they tell you?

SR: About what?

JM: Oh, I don't know! What it's like in the next world? In Heaven?

SR: *[Smiles]* They tell me it's sort of like this one but different. They say that what you think makes everything.

JM: I don't understand.

SR: I don't either, but that's what they say!

JM: What do they mostly talk about?

SR: It depends! Some are happy. Some are at peace. Some worry over their past. Some worry over their family. I have to ignore it sometimes. When they know you can hear them, they'll try to talk till you're blue in the face.

JM: Is it hard to turn it off?

SR: It just takes practice . . . like everything else in this life.

All too soon, I had to leave and get back to Charlottesville. Sadly, I never brought up this topic again. I have spoken with others over the years who communicate with spirit entities, and they tend to echo Mrs. Ramsey's assessment of this form of communication. It appears that Lee Gandee was correct in asserting that spirits are, for the most part, just like you and me—concerned and consumed with their own rather mundane affairs. With the exception of those who are seeking some sort of justice for a wrong done to them, they seem to be occupying a parallel space and time, each immersed in their own state of consciousness, their own awareness and, some would say, their own illusions. Based on most accounts I have heard over the years, unless you really enjoy immersing yourself in other people's lives, the majority of spirit contact is pretty dull. I am, of course, referring to those spirit entities that had been living human lives. Other spirit entities, such as fairies and elementals, are another matter altogether.

During our last visit, I decided to ask Mrs. Ramsey about what she thought about her life.

JM: Mrs. Ramsey, how do you feel about the life you've had?

SR: I'm happy. I don't have any regrets. I'm at peace with the Lord.

JM: What has all of your healing experience done for you?

SR: I don't know what you're asking.

JM: I'm sorry; it's just that you have healed people, delivered babies, even fought with evil. What does all that mean to you?

SR: That my Jesus is everywhere. No matter what happens, He is with me. He's loved me and has blessed me through all my troubles. Now I look forward to going home to be with Him one day soon.

MM: Oh, Grandma, don't talk like that!

SR: But it's true. This old body, it is about used up like an old, worn-out dress. I'm not worried, because one day I'll have a new one to wear in Heaven.

I found myself a bit overwhelmed by her statement, as I knew I was in the presence of a holy person. Simple, decent and magically empowered by her inner faith. She noticed my expression.

SR: Oh, now, that's enough of that. Let's get you some iced tea!

Postscript

The presence of true and unswerving holiness is a blessing to all who can experience it. Perhaps the reason that it has this effect is that a holy person's presence provides a glimpse of the wonderful truth that is behind this often confusing, irritating and mundane world. I always find it creates longing for the presence of the Divine, like a love for its beloved. It is far more powerful than the gaudy and flashy way that some religious people present themselves. For all the noise and verbiage, they cannot hold a candle next to this one Virginian, a small-town, country saint. I will always be grateful to have spent a little time in her presence.

I soon found myself consumed with my studies, my new girlfriend and the promise of a trip abroad. For several years, I sent holiday cards, and one year my card came back with a note from Mary that her grandmother had passed away suddenly in her sleep. She said her grandmother always spoke kindly of me and sometimes asked about me. After a good cry, I realized there was no need to worry. As the old song says, "we'll meet again some day."

Epilogue

Most people are other people. Their thoughts are someone else's opinions, their lives a mimicry, their passions a quotation.

—Oscar Wilde (1854–1900)

We are all priestesses and priests. We are priests and priestesses when we facilitate the spirit or Divine presence and allow it to flow in and through ourselves and others . . . through ritual in church, in magical circle and in everyday life.

—Conversation with a personal friend, Nashville, 2000

I HOPE YOU HAVE ENJOYED the stories of my experiences with American shamanic healers. They have made a lasting impression and impact on my life that has been so enriching, I hardly have the words to describe it. If I have succeeded, perhaps my stories have opened a window for you and given you a glimpse of a world that you may not have known existed or believed was a relic of the distant past. I have tried to share with you what I call a "glimpse of possibility." This glimpse of possibility is the awareness that your world and sense of reality is so much more than you might have thought of before.

Over the years, people have asked me if I thought these old traditions constituted a spiritual path or were just a collection of folk superstitions, practices and remedies. I always answer that I believe there are elements within these traditions that are spiritual. These spiritual elements can open and expand your perception and cause you to see the world in a different way.

Others have asked me to try to be an advocate for their spiritual tradition, based on some connection with one folk religion or other. I cannot and will not, at this age, be a mouthpiece for anyone else's view of spirituality, mysticism or a magically based life. Everyone's spiritual path is their own responsibility, and I am not an advocate for a particular group or tradition.

If this old, magically-based spiritual path is not to fall into a trap, as have other spiritual traditions, its old and new adherents must not, beyond a very limited degree, attempt to codify, organize and structure the mystical experience that is at the heart of the shamanic experience. This is probably the most important message I can give you: Keep this practice a simple, direct path to communication with the Divine. As a musician once said to me, "When you listen to music, just listen, 'cause the minute you start thinking about what you are hearing, you're not listening anymore." Have I got it all figured out? Hardly, but this path has taken me on a wonderful voyage of discovery that continues to this day.

Your spirituality in this life, hopefully, will be an authentic journey of self-discovery and intimate revelation. It is your unique personal expression and search for meaning. It is yours alone. Do not give it away easily to anyone—you have everything you need to fully realize the Divine and the magic in your life, right here, right now, within you. While you may seek guidance from someone or within a particular tradition, in the end, only you can teach yourself. Do not allow anyone or any tradition to mold you beyond the initial information-gathering stage. This hurts you and the other person and stunts the spiritual evolvement of anyone else involved. Others can, at best, only point you in a direction. You must then have the courage and tenacity to continue to follow that direction and grow yourself spiritually.

Authentic spiritual growth takes considerable time and effort, but the rewards are indescribably wonderful. Beware of the easy answers, the charismatic leaders and the flashy presentations. Spirituality is a gradual process of evolving awareness of the Divine and its relation to you and who you believe yourself to be in this life. There will be disappointments and surprises, but you must learn to trust yourself—your true self. Churches, associations and other religious groups can be wonderfully supportive, and we all need them to a degree, but as my late father said, "You entered this world by yourself and you will leave the same way." Don't let others live your spiritual life for you. I can't think of any greater waste of time.

To me, the appeal of the Powwow, Granny-woman and Hoodoo traditions is not only that they are solitary in nature, but that they also are concerned with everyday issues of health, life and death. There are other spiritual benefits, as well. These practices and beliefs allow you to let go of the bounds of your controlled existence and to let yourself feel—to allow you to reach beyond your normal range of consciousness and to welcome the inherent flow of joy that courses through you and out into the world.

I believe that in this life we all have, to varying degrees, the desire to find a path for our soul or spirit. In some cases, we have received a definable calling that drives our real spiritual needs. In recent years, scholars have written extensively about what is called your "spiritual personality." An example is *Soultypes: Decode Your Spiritual DNA to Create a Life of Authenticity, Joy and Grace, by* Robert Norton and Richard Southern. Apparently, each of us has an innate manner in which we respond to the spiritual aspect of our life, and each spiritual personality has a distinct set of spiritual needs.

Some churches use tests that resemble the Myers-Briggs Type Indicator (MBTI) personality tests to determine the spiritual types and needs of their leadership. In this way, by identifying and understanding their basic spiritual personality, individuals can more easily realize and become aware of their spiritual identity and needs. This identification also helps with the management of interpersonal relationships and the group dynamics of a congregation. I have taken this test in a church setting and discovered the following personality types:

The Theologian: This person needs and likes to read, study and discuss religious texts. This is a spiritual path of cognition. This spiritual personality type loves to be in a theological discussion group and often provides excellent analysis of the major tenets of dogma.

The Visionary: This person is motivated by causes, is goal- and project-oriented. This is a spiritual path of action, and this spiritual personality type enjoys social action and community projects and building new church buildings.

The Connector: This individual needs to connect personally and spiritually with others. This is a path of human interaction and communal sharing.

This spiritual personality thrives on periods of fellowship, church suppers and prayer meetings, where joys and concerns can be expressed.

The Mystic: This person yearns personally for intimate, direct encounters with the Divine. This is a path of contemplation, deep, personal searching and often, ecstatic experience. This spiritual personality needs to spend long hours at prayer, take spiritual retreats and be encouraged to write about spiritual encounters. The Mystic often does not fit well into contemporary churches, although some denominations are trying to reach out and appreciate what this person can offer.

Most people fall somewhere in the middle of these personalities, which include traits from the others. This is perfectly normal. In the spiritual life of a community, all of these spiritual personality types are essential, and each makes a valuable contribution. In case you are wondering, when I took the test, I was shown to be profoundly Mystic with a few Connector and Visionary traits. I found this very useful in understanding why this shamanic path has appealed to me and why some things like theological discussions have always been an ordeal to endure.

In Ohio, at spiritual retreat in 2000, I was told by a Unitarian Universalist church leader, "You will never be totally happy with conventional church activities, but we still need you to write and tell us what you experience." It was at that moment that I began the journey of writing this book.

Whatever our spiritual personality type, we must never allow ourselves to accept anything spiritual that *almost* meets our needs or that someone tells us should be adequate. The world's religious communities are full of many good, sincere, spiritually evolved people who can help you—to the limits of their experience. Beware, however, of ego-trippers, control freaks, shysters, deluded and insane people, outright frauds and even well-meaning psychic vampires who will suck away your spiritual strength and leave you spiritually empty.

You must be very careful who you trust. I do not expect you to take my words or experiences as correct or authentic, just because you have read this book. Give yourself permission to experience, to question, to challenge, to explore, to get fooled and temporarily deluded and to uncover the illusions of the frauds and charlatans. Learn to recognize and trust the small, inner voice within you. You will learn and grow with each encounter. Are there dangers on this path? Of course! Is the shamanic path for everyone? Clearly not! Only you can know if you are drawn to do this, and only you will know how far to proceed along this path.

For me, the shaman's path is an approach to my intense need for mystical experience, which I define as a search for a direct personal experience of the Divine. For me, this is a path of union and reunion that has had no parallel in this life of embodied existence. The acts of healing, if persistently and sincerely pursued, are acts of faith that offer a glimpse of that unique Divine experience. After all, if you can open yourself enough to allow the Divine to move through your physical form, are you not healed as well?

Pain and sickness of all kinds are hints, reminders to us that this world and our physical forms are temporary and insubstantial. We are happy, then sad; feel joy and then are destined to suffer again. Where is the satisfaction in such a circular process?

Jesus of Nazareth advised us to seek first the Kingdom of God and all things would be added thereafter. I believe the Divine in this particular form was advising us to keep at least a part of our awareness focused on what is lasting, while acknowledging that we all have to continue our time in this embodied state.

The skill of the modern shaman comes from learning to live within this chaotic world, with the ability to consciously shift perceptions and views of reality when needed—and still provide for the needs of daily life. In all likelihood, no group in this culture is going to financially sponsor your spiritual efforts, so you have an additional challenge to your shamanistic practice. Actually, such a challenge is valuable, as it will keep you personally and emotionally anchored as you develop your inner awareness.

We all deeply long for and grieve the loss of our mundane associations and possessions, but how many of us feel the agony of our separation from the Divine enough to earnestly yearn for it? How many of us feel ill at the absence of the Divine's presence? We may chase all manner of illusions and create all manner of theologies, devils and inner ghosts, which only leave us hungry again in a short while. St. Teresa of Avila said, "All things are passing, God never changes. . . . God alone suffices." If you earnestly and unselfconsciously pursue the healing power of communion with the Divine, you will not be denied.

Recently I was talking to a friend and wise-woman, someone I truly respect, about the concepts of the priesthood and of magic. She listened for a while and finally said, "Jack, after all these years we've spent together, you should know by now: We are all priestesses and priests. We are priests and priestesses when we facilitate the spirit or Divine presence and allow it to flow in and through ourselves and others through ritual in church, in magical circle and in everyday life. When we prepare a meal that brings joy to our family and friends, we make magic. When we listen and witness to each other's joys and concerns, we make magic. When we dance and sing in uncontrolled joy and help others to find this experience, we make magic. You may make rules to guide you, but that's the only reason they exist. Authentic spirituality or faith is about letting go, not holding on, because without an authentic intimate, personal spiritual experience, no matter how well a ritual is performed or a sermon is delivered, it is lifeless and worthless." Rituals and sermons are merely vehicles for an inner transformation of your personal view of reality.

In conclusion, I hope my own experiences will offer you ideas and practices that will be useful in your spiritual quest. I hope that you will be the one to create your own magic, to start to weave your own life story and to participate in your own form of healing, whatever your religious tradition or spiritual practice. In this way, you will be reawakening to the infinite moment, that exquisite source of joy that is always at the core of your being. You have always been a work in progress, just like the universe itself.

May you journey well and find that which you seek.

Powwow Charms

THE CREATION AND USE OF CHARMS has been an essential part of an American shaman's practice. Charms, in this sense, are not the costume jewelry version of faddish practice, but a series of natural and manmade objects that are charged with personal psychic energy to perform a certain magical assignment. The process of charging involves the transference of one's personal energy to into a created object. Lee Gandee called this process magnetization, because its purpose is to infuse or magically "magnetize" an object with your energy. Magnetizing requires the same sort of empathic merging that occurs when a Powwow enters the client's psychic realm as part of the healing or during the tracing of a person's energy residues or trails.

Common Powwow charms that I came across in my research included the following:

Charm Bag: A small bag containing herbs and other objects, such as a lodestone. This type of charm is identical to the type given by Hoodoo and Appalachian healers. Traditionally, a charm of this type is worn about the neck and used to ward off evil and illness. It contains asafetida/Ferula asafetida, a pungent, vile-smelling plant resin. Lee once said to me, "No spirit in his right mind would go near something that smelled like that!"

Holey Stones: A naturally occurring amulet was a Holey, Holed, Odin or Hag stone. Art historian Chris Whitcombe's website, Earth Mysteries, has a short article called "Healing Stones," and the website The Stone Pages: Stones of England, "Mên-an-Tol: Standing Stones: Cornwall" provide intriguing glimpses into beliefs about these stones (for more information see the Bibliography.) Whitcombe writes:

Healing properties were especially associated with stones with holes in them. The most famous example is Mên-an-Tol, also known as the Crick Stone, near Madron in Cornwall. According to an 18th-century source, sufferers from pains in the back and limbs were cured after crawling through the hole in his boulder-sized stone. Also, children suffering from rickets (a disease of infancy and childhood characterized by defective bone growth caused by a lack of vitamin D in the body) or a crick in the neck would be cured after being passed three or nine times through the hole, usually against the sun (widdershins). For the cure to work, it was important that boys were passed from a woman to a man, and girls from a man to a woman. ("Healing Stones" par.4)

The smaller wearable versions of Holey Stones are believed to offer protection from magical intrusions, have healing properties and provide, under the proper circumstances, a porthole to view the spirit world.

Bellarmine or Witch Bottle: A bottle that is filled with various herbs, objects, and often something personal, such as hair, fingernails or even blood or urine. These magical objects are placed somewhere in or around the client's dwelling to protect or curse a person or family. For protection, bellarmines are most often positioned in a chimney or under an entrance, such as a door. On occasion, they could be employed to trap and secure a malevolent spirit. Reporter Greig Watson writes in the BBC News online article "Artefact Recalls Witches' Shadow" that a witch bottle was recently discovered in England, near Lincolnshire, in the village of Navenby. The witch bottle was dated to 1830 and, in general, described as, "bent pins, human hair and perhaps urine, the bottles were supposed to protect a household against evil spells" (Watson par. 2).

Written Charms: Many charms contain at least one piece of paper with either names or certain magical symbols or formula inscribed upon it. Three commonly used formulas are described below.

Abracadabra: Daniel Stuhlman's online essay on Abracadabra on the Librarian's Lobby website lists a few possible origins for the word:

It was first mentioned in a poem by Quintus Serenus Sammonicus in the second century. It is believed to have come into English via French from a Greek word abrasadabra (the change from s to c seems to have been through a confused transliteration of the Greek). It originated as a secret and mystical word with a Gnostic sect in Alexandria called the Basilidians (named after their founder Basilides of Egypt). The word was possibly based on Abrasax, the name of an Egyptian deity. It was used as charm to cure toothaches and infectious diseases. The word Abrasax was said to have magical powers. Using the gematria [1] of the Greek letters the holy names Abraxas (Ἀβραξάς) and Mithras (Μίθρας) the Gnostics equated the numerical values of 365, the days of the year. Because of the relationship of Abraxas to the number of days, it was frequently used on amulets and precious stones. (par. 4)

```
A
A B
A B R
A B R A
A B R A C
A B R A C A
A B R A C A D
A B R A C A D A
A B R A C A D A B
A B R A C A D A B R
A B R A C A D A B R A
```

The *Sator Rotas Opera* palindrome is another formula of ancient origin written as a 5-line square:

```
S A T O R
A R E P O
T E N E T
O P E R A
R O T A S
```

The earliest version of this square was found on the wall of a house in the ill-fated city of Pompeii and dates to around 79 A.D. This information comes from Eliot Marshal Smith's website Smithtrust.com:

Although used by early Christian Mystics as a magical charm the square has surfaced in cultures and religions all over the world. Because of the hidden anagram, Pater Noster, The square was originally thought to be of Christian design, but there is now strong evidence that it predates Christianity by a considerable margin and refers to the ancient God, Mithras. (Smith par.1)

According to John George Hohman's *Long Lost Friend,* it is also used for the extinguishing of a fire when water is not available.

Himmelsbrief: A third type of written charm is known as the *Himmelsbrief* or Heavenly Letter, supposedly written to mankind from heaven. The text of the letter is a prayer, combined with verses from the Bible, which promises protection to the bearer from death and injury. *Himmelsbrief* are said to date back to the 16th century and the Thirty Years War. I never encountered one in the Dutch Fork but was informed that American soldiers in the First World War from the Fork carried them. Modern Pennsylvania Hexenmeister Karl Herr reminds us that "writing a Himmelsbrief is casting a spell" (96) and "the most important part is the mental concentration and care you use when you are writing out a Himmelsbrief" (96). Herr has created *Himmelsbrief* for a variety of requests, including protecting his client from the torments of a deceased relative. Here is that *Himmelsbrief:*

> As Christ commanded that the dead should bury the dead, in his name I tell (name) that she must remain here in patient waiting until our Lord comes in glory for her judgment. I pray that our Lord let her not attempt to walk abroad, let her not trouble the living, and let her not disturb those whom she knew in life in any way. In the name of Jesus Christ, the savior and redeemer of us all. Amen. (100)

Please note that most traditional *Himmelsbrief* are too long to present an example but several are available on the Internet.

Many common household items are employed for magical purposes. Here are just a few examples:

Table Salt: Used primarily as a protective barrier or to secure an area. Lee taught me to place salt in a line across a windowsill or doorway to prevent entry by unseen entities. The salt apparently burns their more subtle forms. Salt is also used for the same purpose in Hoodoo, suggesting the cross-cultural natural of many traditions.

Iron: In the form of an iron rod or horseshoe with the open end turned upward towards the ceiling. The iron will diffuse any psychic energy into the air.

Silver: In the form of money or jewelry, silver should be worn or carried on one's person at all times. Should the silver tarnish suddenly or overnight, this is an indication that someone is projecting negative energy toward you. Once you have sought protection, the blackened silver should then be cleaned with brick dust.

Water: Universally, water is used for a variety of magical purposes, including healing and dispelling evil influences from a person. Lee taught me that if I felt myself under attack from an invisible force, to quickly splash water over my face and neck, then wash my hands thoroughly. Spirit energy cannot sustain itself in rain nor can a spell be cast during a storm.

Mirrors: Used for scrying and other divinatory purposes, including spirit contact.

Spoken Powwow Charms and a Physical Charm for Protection against Bad Hexes or Magical Intrusions

Noted here are several traditional spoken Powwow charms for various common ailments. The symbols + + + refer to making the sign of the cross three times in sequence.

For Bleeding:

A. Jesus Christ, Dearest Blood that stoppeth this pain that stoppeth this blood, until The Virgin Mary bring forth another son. Thy womb recreates the world again. In the name of the Father, the Son, and the Holy Ghost.

B. And when I passed by thee and saw thee polluted in thine own blood, I said unto thee when thou wast in thy blood, Live; yea, I said unto thee when thou wast in thy blood, Live.

C. This is the day on which the injury happened. Blood, thou must stop, until the Virgin Mary bring forth another son. Repeat these words three times.

For Burns:

A. Burn, burn, I blow on thee, in the name of the Father, the Son
   and the Holy Ghost.

B. Three holy men went out walking,
   They did bless the heat and the burning;
   They blessed that it might not increase;
   They blessed that it might quickly cease! + + +

For Bruises and swelling injuries:

A. Bruise, thou shalt not heat;
   Bruise, thou shalt not sweat;
   Bruise, thou shalt not run,
   No-more than Virgin Mary shall bring forth another son. + + +

B. Three pure virgins went out on a journey to inspect a swelling
   and sickness. The first one said, "It is hoarse." The second said, "It
   is not." The third said, "If it is not, then will our Lord Jesus Christ
   come." This must be spoken in the name of the Holy Trinity.

To take pain from a wound:

Cut three small twigs from a tree—each to be cut off in one cut
—stroke one end of each twig in the wound, and wrap them separately
in a piece of white paper, and put them in a warm and dry place.

A Charm for Psychic Protection

There are nine primary ingredients and nine steps in the assembling of this
charm. The number nine is sacred to the art of Powwow, as it is three times
three (3 x 3). Three is sacred to the three holy names (see below). The total
number of ingredients and steps is 18 or crunched is 9. Number symbolism is very important in Powwow spellwork, as it help to focus the human
energy that energizes the charm and casts the spell, which, in this case, is
called a prayer. The bag itself is considered a manifestation of that prayer.
The reader will notice ingredients used that are also common to Hoodoo.
The holy names may be modified for those of other faiths. All holy names
work equally well.

Ingredients: Note that there are nine basic ingredients.

1. One small red flannel bag (you can make your own if you like)

2. One piece of unlined, white paper—letter stock (1.5 inches x 1.5 inches)

3. One small lodestone (for energizing the charm)

4. Three small pinches of vervain root (protection against evil energy in spirit form)

5. One small (half-inch) piece of Orris root (protection against negative but passive human energy)

6. One small (half-inch) piece of High John Conqueror Root (protects against bad witchcraft or ritually produced energy/spellwork)

7. One small piece of red thread (6 inches long) to tie the scroll

8. One dram of Van Van Oil (commonly known as the herb lemongrass) or magnetic oil (to "dress" or bring the powers sleeping in the two roots to life. You only need three drops for each root.)

9. One red candle (to seal the scroll and the charm)

Preparing the charm: Note that there are nine steps in this process.

1. Prepare yourself to produce this charm by taking a salt bath with vinegar or lemon. Clear your mind of daily distractions as you enter a semi-trance state (shamanic awareness).

2. Secure your environment from psychic forces by creating a circle of salt, sprinkling of holy water or placing iron implements to protect the area.

3. Dress the Orris and High John Conqueror roots: Put three drops of the Van Van oil in your left palm, place each root in the oil and coat each root by rubbing the oil onto it with your right thumb as you chant:

Lord Jesus Christ, hear my plea,
Protect (name) from harm and set (him/her) free.

(Repeat this process for each root and place them in the bag)

4. Place three small pinches of vervain in the bag as you chant:

Sacred herb, from Mary's breast,
Protect (name) and give (her/him) rest.

5. Rub the lodestone with the oil and chant:

Stone that attracts, and repulses, too,
Protect this soul, (name), I ask of you.

Place the stone into the bag.

6. When preparing a charm for someone, you must individualize the charm by using an item from their person, such as a small lock of hair or fingernail parings; even a drop of blood. If this is a charm you are preparing for yourself, you should do the same; note that blood is especially significant when creating a charm for your own personal protection. Take all sanitary precautions when handling blood.

7. On the piece of unlined letter-stock paper, carefully write in black or red ink the following:

I.

N. I. R.

I.

SANCTUS   SPIRITUS

I.

N. I. R.

I.

ALL THIS BE GUARDED HEREIN TIME, AND THERE IN ETER-
NITY. AMEN.

8. Roll the paper into a scroll, then tie the red thread around it using three knots. Place tied scroll into the bag. Light the red candle and seal the knot with three drops of wax as you say:

With this wax I bind this charm,
I seal this prayer, to keep (name) from harm.

9. Close the bag and wrap it securely by tying the drawstrings in three
   knots. Then seal the knots with nine drops of wax as you say:

With this wax I bind this charm,
I seal this prayer, to keep (name) from harm,
In the name of the Father, Son and Holy Ghost.
AMEN.

To finish the charm, I usually pray/chant a short personal prayer over
the bag nine times, three times each day for three days, for the relief and
protection of the person for whom I have made the charm. I leave the
charm on my altar, where I keep it in a plastic bag or envelope to avoid
contamination by other energies, until I place it in the person's hands, at
which point I say, "From my hand to yours, be at peace." You may place
the charm where you normally do your magical work for three days before
delivering it to the one for whom it was created.

Again please note the importance of the numbers in the spell-work:

9 Ingredients + 9 steps + 9 finishing prayers = 27, which reduces to
$$2 + 7 = 9$$

All things in Powwow spiritually cycle back to recognition of the ultimate, yet intimate role that the Divine plays in our lives and in the eternal
cycle of existence.

You now know how to make a Powwow charm of protection. This is
the first time I have passed this on to others since this spell was passed on
to me by Lee Gandee almost thirty years ago.

Bibliography

Preface

Goldberg, Myshele. "What's in a Name? Colonial Dynamics in Spiritual Practice." *PanGaia* 46 (2007): 23-24.

Hawkins, John. "Magical Medical Practice in South Carolina." *Popular Science Monthly* 70 (Feb. 1907): 164-74 (Reprint).

Mayo, Katherine. *Mother India.* New York: Harcourt, Brace & Co, 1927.

Introduction: What Is Magic? What Are Magical Healings and Shamanism?

Aldhouse-Green, Miranda and Stephen Aldhouse-Green. *The Quest of the Shaman: Shape-Shifters, Sorcerers and Spirit-Healers of Ancient Europe.* London: Thames and Hudson, 2005.

Brady, Erika. "Bad Scares and Joyful Hauntings: 'Priesting': The Supernatural Predicament." *Out of the Ordinary: Folklore and the Supernatural.* Ed. Barbara Walker. Logan, Utah: Utah State University Press, 1995. 145-57.

Hand, Wayland D. *Magical Medicine: The Folkloric Component of Medicine in the Folk Belief, Custom and Ritual of the Peoples of Europe and America.* Berkeley: University of California Press, 1980.

Harner, Michael. "Science, Spirits, and Core Shamanism." *Shamanism* 12.1 (Spring/Summer 1999). 14 July 2007 *http://www.shamanism.org/articles/article10.html.*

Harner, Michael. *The Way of the Shaman.* New York, Harper and Row, 1980.

Hohman, Johann Georg. *John George Hohman's Pow-Wows, or, Long Lost Friend: A Collection of Mysterious and Invaluable Arts and Remedies for Man As Well As Animals; with Many Proofs of Their Virtue and Efficacy in Healing Diseases, Etc., the Greater Part of Which Was Never Published Until They Appeared in Print for the First Time in the U.S. in 1820.* Pomeroy, WA: Health Research, 1971.

Horrigan, Bonnie. "Shamanic Healing: We Are Not Alone: An Interview of Michael Harner." *Shamanism* 10.1 (Spring-Summer 1997). 14 July 2007 <http://www.shamanism.org/articles/article01.html>.

Hufford, David J. "Beings without Bodies: An Experience-Centered Theory of the Belief in Spirits." *Out of the Ordinary: Folklore and the Supernatural.* Ed. Barbara Walker. Logan, Utah: Utah State University Press, 1995. 11-45.

Kalweit, Holger. *Shamans, Healers and Medicine Men.* Boston: Shambhala, 2001.

McClenon, James. "Supernatural Experience, Folk Belief and Spiritual Healing." Ed. Barbara Walker. *Out of the Ordinary: Folklore and the Supernatural.* Logan, Utah: Utah State University Press, 1995. 107-21.

Walsh, Roger N. *The Spirit of Shamanism.* New York: J.P. Putnam's Sons, 1990.

Yoder, Don. "Toward A Definition of Folk Religion." *Western Folklore* 33 (1974): 14.

Chapter One

Adams, Dennis, and Hillary Barnwell. "The Gullah Language and Sea Island Culture, Part II: The Sea Island Culture: Religion." 2004. *Beaufort County Public Library*. 08 August 2007 <http://www.beaufortcountylibrary.org/rooms/documents/html/gullah2.htm#Religion>.

Bailey, Cornelia Walker. *God, Dr. Buzzard and the Bolito Man: A Saltwater Geechee Talks about Life on Sapelo Island*. Georgia. New York: Anchor Books, 2000.

Beaufort County (SC) Library. "Famous People of Beaufort County, SC." 2 Jan. 2007. *Beaufort County (SC) Library*. 14 July 2007 <http://www.beaufortcountylibrary.org/rooms/documents/html/famous.htm>.

Chicora Foundation. "The Lives of African-American Slaves in Carolina during the Eighteenth Century." Understanding Slavery: The Lives of Eighteenth Century African-Americans. 1996. *SCIway.net*. 14 July 2007 <http://www.sciway.net/hist/chicora/slavery18-3.html>.

Chireau, Yvonne P. *Black Magic: Religion and the African American Conjuring Tradition*. Berkeley: University of California Press, 2003.

Dean, Will. "Hoodoo Medicine in the Lowcountry." *Lowcountry Now* (March 7, 2004). 14 July 2007 <http://www.lowcountrynow.com/stories/030704/LOChoodoo.shtml>.

Floyd, E. Randall. "Plat-Eye Thought to Be Ghost of Deceased." 15 Dec. 1996. *Augusta Chronicle Online:* Features @ Augusta. 14 July 2007 <http://chronicle.augusta.com/stories/121596/floyd.html>.

Frazer, James Gordon. "Sympathetic Magic." *The Golden Bough: A Study in Magic and Religion*. New York: Macmillan, 1922. *Bartleby.com: Great Books Online*. 08 August 2007 <http://www.bartleby.com/196/5.html>.

———. "Contagious Magic." *The Golden Bough: A Study in Magic and Religion*. New York: Macmillan, 1922. *Bartleby.com: Great Books Online*. 08 August 2007 <http://www.bartleby.com/196/7.html>.

"From Indentured Servitude to Racial Slavery." *Africans in America: The Terrible Transformation*, Part 1: 1450-1750. PBS. WGBH, Boston.1999. 08 August 2007 <http://www.pbs.org/wgbh/aia/part1/1narr3.html>.

Hohman, Johann Georg. *John George Hohman's Pow-Wows, or, Long Lost Friend: A Collection of Mysterious and Invaluable Arts and Remedies for Man As Well As Animals; with Many Proofs of Their Virtue and Efficacy in Healing Diseases, Etc., the Greater Part of Which Was Never Published Until They Appeared in Print for the First Time in the U.S. in 1820*. Pomeroy, WA: Health Research, 1971.

Hyatt, Harry Middleton. *Hoodoo—Conjuration—Witchcraft—Rootwork; Beliefs Accepted by Many Negroes and White Persons, These Being Orally Recorded Among Blacks and Whites*. [Hannibal, Mo: Printed by Western Pub.; distributed by American University Bookstore, Washington, 1970.]

Johnson, F. Roy. *The Fabled Doctor Jim Jordan; A Story of Conjure*. [Murfreesboro, N. C.: Johnson, 1963.]

Long, Carolyn Morrow. *Spiritual Merchants: Religion, Magic and Commerce*. Knoxville, TN: University of Tennessee Press, 2001.

McColley, Robert. "Virginia, Slavery in." *Dictionary of Afro-American Slavery*. New York: Greenwood Press, 1988.

McTeer, J. E. *High Sheriff of the Low Country*. Beaufort, S.C.: Beaufort Book Co, 1970.

Matthews, Holly F. "Doctors and Root Doctors: Patients Who Use Both." *Herbal and Magical Medicine: Traditional Healing Today*. Ed. James Kirdland. Durham: Duke University Press, 1992.

Michaelson, Mike. "Can A 'Root Doctor' Actually Put A Hex on or Is It All A Great Put-on?" *Today's Health* 39:42 (March 1972).

Mitchell, Faith. *Hoodoo Medicine: Gullah Herbal Remedies*. Columbia, S.C.: Summerhouse Press, 1999.

Olwell, Robert. *Masters, Slaves and Subjects: The Culture of Power in the South Carolina Low Country, 1740–1790*. Ithaca: Cornell University Press, 1998.

Pinckney, Roger. *Blue Roots: African-American Folk Magic of the Gullah People*. St. Paul: Llewellyn Publications, 1998.

Pollitzer, William S. *The Gullah People and their African Heritage*. Athens: University of Georgia Press, 1999.

Puckett, Newbell Niles. *Folk Beliefs of the Southern Negro*. New York: Dover Publications, 1969 (Reprint).

Talty, Stephan. "Spooked: The White Slave Narratives, *Transition* 10.1 (2000): 48-75.

Tannenbaum, Frank. *Slave and Citizen: The Negro in the Americas*. New York: A. A. Knopf, 1947.

Watson, Wilbur. *Black Folk Medicine: The Therapeutic Significance of Faith and Trust*. Transaction Books: New Brunswick: Transaction Books, 1984.

Yronwode, Catherine. "Hoodoo: African American Magic." Hoodoo in Theory and Practice. 2003. *Lucky Mojo Curio Company*. 08 August 2007 <http://www.luckymojo.com/hoodoohistory.html>.

———. *Hoodoo Herb and Root Magic: A Materia Magica of African-American Conjure and Traditional Formulary, Giving the Spiritual Uses of Natural Herbs, Roots, Minerals, and Zoological Curios*. Forestville, Calif: Lucky Mojo Curio Co, 2002.

Chapter Two

McTeer, J. E. *High Sheriff of the Low Country*. Beaufort, S.C.: Beaufort Book Co, 1970.

Davis, Rod. *American Voudou: Journey into a Hidden World*, rev. ed. Denton, TX: University of North Texas Press, 1999.

Chapter Three

Bernheim, G. D. *History of the German Settlements and of the Lutheran Church in North and South Carolina, from the Earliest Period of the Colonization of the Dutch, German, and Swiss Settlers to the Close of the First Half of the Present Century*. Spartanburg, South Carolina: The Reprint Company, 1974.

Boyer, Dennis. "Braucher's Progress: A Preliminary Reevaluation of Pennsylvania German Folk Medicine." *Newsletter of the Friends of the Max Kade Institute* 8.4 (Winter 1999). 08 August 2007 <http://csumc.wisc.edu/mki/Newsletter/newsw00.html#braucher>.

Ellisor, Vickie. "More Interesting Tales: 'Was She a Witch or Not?'" Believe it or Not: South Carolina Folklore. 17 September 2007. <http://www.palmettoroots.org/SCFolklore.html>

Gandee, Lee R. *Strange Experience: The Secrets of A Hexenmeister: How to Employ the Hex Signs and Spoken Spells of Rural American Folk Magic.* Englewood Cliffs, NJ: Prentice-Hall, Inc., 1971.

Gandee, Lee. "Using" to Heal in South Carolina." *Fate Magazine* (March 1961): 34-39.

Hawkins, John. "Magical Medical Practice in South Carolina." *Popular Science Monthly* 70 (Feb. 1907): 164-74 (Reprint).

Hershberger, Jacob J. and Effie Troyer. "Healing Charms." *Amish Roots: A Treasury of History, Wisdom and Lore. Amish Roots: A Treasury of History, Wisdom and Lore.* Ed. John A. Hostetler. Baltimore: Johns Hopkins University Press, 1989.

Hollis, Daniel W. *History of St. Andrews and the Dutch Fork.* Columbia, S.C.: Home Federal Savings and Loan, n.d.

Jordan, Mildred. *The Distelfink Country of the Pennsylvania Dutch.* New York: Crown Publishers, 1978.

Korson, George. *Black Rock: Mining Folklore of the Pennsylvania Dutch.* Baltimore: The Johns Hopkins Press, 1960.

Kriebel, David. "Powwowing: A Persistent Healing Tradition." *Pennsylvania German Review* (Fall 2001): 14-22. 16 July 2007 <http://www.kutztown.edu/community/pgchc/hcn/german_review.pdf>.

Milspaw, Yvonne J. "Witchcraft Belief in a Pennsylvania German Family." *Pennsylvania Folklife* 27.4 (1978): 14-31.

O'Neall, John Belton, and John Abney Chapman. *The Annals of Newberry: in Two Parts.* Newberry, S.C.: Aull & Houseal, 1892.

Reed, Brenda Helen Keck. "Henry Melchior Muhlenberg's Journal Account of the Weberite Cult (1759-1761) at Saxe Gotha, South Carolina." 16 April 2005. *The Weberite Heresy & Murders: Myth, Madness, & Murder in the Colony of South Carolina.* 14 July 2007 <http://www.homestead.com/weberites/>.

Reimensnyder, Barbara L. *Powwowing in Union County: A Study of Pennsylvania German Folk Medicine in Context.* New York, NY: AMS Press, 1989.

Sachse, Julius Friedrich. *The German Pietists of Provincial Pennsylvania, 1694-1708.* New York: AMS Press, 1970.

Walker, Marlene Koon. "Did you hear about . . .'using' in South Carolina?" *Believe it or Not: South Carolina Heresies, Folklore, Shocking Revelations, Murder, Mayhem & Mystery.* Excerpted from Bayne, Coy. *Lake Murray: Legend and Leisure,* 2nd ed. Sunset, S.C.: Bayne Pub. Co, 1992. 17 September 2007 <http://www.palmettoroots.org/SC_Believe_It_Or_Not.html>

"The Witch Murder Verdicts." *Literary Digest* (January 26, 1929): 11.

Chapter Four

Albertus. *Albertus Magnus; Being the Approved, Verified, Sympathetic and Natural Egyptian Secrets; or, White and Black Art for Man and Beast. The Book of Nature and Hidden Secrets and Mysteries of Life Unveiled; Being the Forbidden Knowledge of Ancient Philosophers.* Translated from the German. Chicago: Egyptian Pub. Co, 1900.

Beissel, William Wilson. *Secrets of Sympathy. Chapbook, 1938. Reprinted in Powwow Power: A True Story of A Powwow Relative and Other Related Events,* By James D. Beissel. Willow Street, PA: Crystal Educational Counselors, 1998.

Canon, Scott. "Amish 'Voodoo' Applies Belief in Healing Power." *Kansas City Star* 20 October 1996: A10.

Dieffenbach, Victor C. "Powwowing Among the Pennsylvania Germans." *Pennsylvania Folklife* 21 (February 1975): 29-46.

Fooks, David. "The History of Hex Signs." *Pennsylvania German Review* (Fall 2001): 12-13.

Frazier, Paul. "Some Lore of Hexing and Powwowing." *Midwest Folklore* (Summer 1952): 101-07.

Gandee, Lee R. *Strange Experience: The Secrets of A Hexenmeister: How to Employ the Hex Signs and Spoken Spells of Rural American Folk Magic.* Englewood Cliffs, NJ: Prentice-Hall, Inc., 1971.

Grimassi, Raven. *Encyclopedia of Wicca & Witchcraft.* St. Paul, MN, Llewellyn Worldwide, 2000.

Hohman, John George. "To Remove Bruises and Pains." *Powwows: or, Long Lost Friend: a collection of mysterious and invaluable arts and remedies, for man as well as animals with many proofs Of their virtue and efficacy in healing diseases, etc., the greatest part which was never published until they appeared in print for the first time in the U.S. in the year 1820.* Internet Sacred Text Archive.14 September 2007 <www.sacred-texts.com/ame/pow/pow042.htm>

Igou, Brad. "The Story of the Hex Sign." *Amish Country News,* October 2001. 14 July 2007 <http://www.amishnews.com/featurearticles/storyofhexsigns.htm>

Kuna, Ralph A. "Hoodoo: The Indigenous Medicine and Psychiatry of the Black American." *Mankind Quarterly* 18.2 (Oct-Dec 1977): 137-51.

Herr, Karl. *Hex and Spellwork: The Magical Practices of the Pennsylvania Dutch.* York Beach, ME: Red Wheel/Weiser, 2002.

Peterson, John H. *Romanus-Büchlein: Vor Gott Der Herr Bewahre Meine Seele, Meinen Aus- Und Eingang; Von Nun An Bis in Alle Ewigkeit, Amen. Halleluja. (Little Book of The Roma, Before God The Lord Preserve My Soul, My Going and Coming; From Now to All Eternity, Amen. Halleluja.).* Venice, 1788. 2006. EsotericArchives.com. 14 July 2007 <http://www.esotericarchives.com/moses/romanus.htm>

Scheible Johann. *The Sixth and Seventh Books of Moses: Moses' Magical Spirit-Art: Known As the Wonderful Arts of the Old Wise Hebrews, Taken from the Mosaic Books of the Cabala and the Talmud for the Good of Mankind.* Escondido, CA: Book Tree, 1999.

"Stovepipe." Personal email correspondence. 1 August 2002.

Yoder, Don. "Hohman and Romanus: Origins and Diffusion of the Pennsylvania German Powwow Manual." Ed. Wayland D. Hand. *American Folk Medicine: A Symposium.* Berkeley: University of California Press. 235-248.

Chapter Five

Budge, E. A. Wallis. *Amulets and Superstitions: The Original Texts with Translations and Descriptions of a Long Series of Egyptian, Sumerian, Assyrian, Hebrew, Christian,*

Gnostic, and Muslim Amulets and Talismans and Magical Figures, with Chapters on the Evil Eye, the Origin of the Amulet, the Pentagon, the Swastika, the Cross (Pagan and Christian), the Properties of Stones, Rings, Divination, Numbers, the Kabbalah, Ancient Astrology, Etc. New York: Dover Publications, 1978.

Grimassi, Raven. *Encyclopedia of Wicca & Witchcraft.* St. Paul, MN, Llewellyn Worldwide, 2000, p. 456.

Hawkins, John. "Magical Medical Practice in South Carolina." *Popular Science Monthly* 70 (Feb. 1907): 164-74 (Reprint).

Hicks, Theresa M. "Did you hear about ...Witchcraft in South Carolina?" *Believe it or not? South Carolina Heresies, Folklore, Shocking Revelations, Murder, Mayhem & Mystery.* 18 September 2007 <http://www.palmettoroots.org/SC_Believe_It_Or_Not.html>

Kibler, James E. *A Carolina Dutch Fork Calendar: Manners and Customs in the Olden Times.* Athens, Ga: Dutch Fork Press, 1988.

Chapter Six

Eliade, Mircea, and Willard R. Trask. *Shamanism: Archaic Techniques of Ecstasy.* Bollingen series, 76. New York: Bollingen Foundation; distributed by Pantheon Books, 1964.

"Jane Roberts." 17 September 2007. *Wikipedia.* 18 September 2007 <http://en.wikipedia.org/wiki/Jane_Roberts>

Roberts, Jane, and Seth. *The Seth Material.* Englewood Cliffs, N.J.: Prentice-Hall, 1970.

Chapter Seven

Hawkins, John. "Magical Medical Practice in South Carolina." *Popular Science Monthly* 70 (Feb. 1907): 164-74 (Reprint).

McClaskey, Thomas R. "Decoding Traumatic Memory Patterns at the Cellular Level." 1998. *The American Academy of Experts in Traumatic Stress,* Inc. 14 July 2007 <http://www.aaets.org/article30.htm>.

MacManus, Diarmuid Arthur. *The Middle Kingdom: The Faerie World of Ireland.* Parrish, 1960.

Simpson, Jacqueline. *The Folklore of Sussex.* London: Batsford, 1973.

Turner, Edith. "The Reality of Spirits." *Shamanism,* 10:1 (Spring/Summer 1997). 08 August 2007. <http://www.shamanism.org/articles/article02.html>.

Chapter Eight

Gandee, Lee R. *Strange Experience: The Secrets of A Hexenmeister: How to Employ the Hex Signs and Spoken Spells of Rural American Folk Magic.* Englewood Cliffs, NJ: Prentice-Hall, Inc., 1971.

Sachse, Julius Friedrich. *The German Pietists of Provincial Pennsylvania, 1694–1708.* New York: AMS Press, 1970.

Chapter Nine

Byrne, Rhonda. *The Secret.* New York: Atria Books, 2006

Flowers, Stephen E. *The Galdrabok: An Icelandic Grimoire.* York Beach, ME: S. Weiser, 1989.

Gandee, Lee R. *Strange Experience: The Secrets of A Hexenmeister: How to Employ the Hex Signs and Spoken Spells of Rural American Folk Magic.* Englewood Cliffs, NJ: Prentice-Hall, Inc., 1971.

Herr, Karl. *Hex and Spellwork: The Magical Practices of the Pennsylvania Dutch.* York Beach, ME: Red Wheel/Weiser, 2002.

Chapter Ten

Brown, Richard Maxwell. *The South Carolina Regulators.* Cambridge, MA: Belknap Press, 1963.

Cavender, Anthony. *Folk Medicine in Southern Appalachia.* Chapel Hill: UNC Press, 2003.

Coggeshall, John M. *Carolina Piedmont Country* (Folklife in the South Series). Jackson MS; University Press of Mississippi, 1996

Davies, Owen. *Cunning-Folk: Popular Magic in English History.* London: Hambledon and London, 2003.

——— and Jack Semmons. "Cunningfolk Gallery: Tamsin Blight [Blee]: Mid-19th Century." *Cunningfolk.Com.* 14 July 2007 <http://www.karisgarden.com/cunningfolk/gallery.htm>.

———. "Charmers and Charming in England and Wales from the Eighteenth to the Twentieth Century." *Folklore* 109 (1998): 41-53.

———. 2006. *Cunningfolk.com:* 14 July 2007 <http://www.karisgarden.com/cunningfolk/home.htm>.

Frome, Michael. *Strangers in High Places: The Story of the Great Smokey Mountains.* Knoxville, TN: University of Tennessee Press, 1980.

Grantham, Paul. "Daddy Witch's Grave: Horseheath, Cambridgeshire." *Paul Grantham; Unconsecrated Burials of Britain.* 08 August 2007. <http://www.grantham.karoo.net/paul/graves/daddy.htm>.

Hole, Christina. *Witchcraft in England.* London: Batsford, 1977.

Jones-Baker, Doris. *The Folklore of Hertfordshire.* Totowa, N.J.: Rowman and Littlefield, 1977.

Kendrick, Sue. "The Cunning Men of Essex." 2005. *Timetravel-Britain.com.* 14 July 2007 <http://www.timetravel-britain.com/05/fall/cunning.shtml>.

Knowles, George. *James "Cunning" Murrell (The Master of Witches).* 03 May 2007. *Controverscial.com.* 16 July 2007. <http://www.controverscial.com/James%20Cunning%20Murrell.htm>.

MacLennan, W. J. "Illness without Doctors: Medieval Systems of Healthcare in Scotland." *Journal of the Royal College of Physicians-Edinburgh* 32.1 (2002): 59-67.

McCoy, Edain. *In a Graveyard at Midnight: Folk Magick and Wisdom from the Heart of Appalachia.* (Llewellyn's Practical Magick series). St. Paul: Llewellyn Publications, 1995.

Moss, Kay K. *Southern Folk Medicine, 1750–1820.* Columbia: University of South Carolina Press, 1999.

Obelkevich, James. *Religion and Rural Society: South Lindsey, 1825–1875.* Oxford: Clarendon Press, 1976.

Rowling, Marjorie. *The Folklore of the Lake District*. Totowa, N.J.: Rowman and Little-field, 1976.

Ryan, Meda. *Biddy Early: [the Wise Woman of Clare]*. Cork: Mercier Press, 1991

Simpson, Jacqueline. *The Folklore of Sussex*. London: Batsford, 1973.

Strivelli, Ginger. "Appalachian Granny Magic." 2001. *Witchvox Traditions*. 14 July 2007 <http://www.witchvox.com/va/dt_va.html?a=usnc&c=trads&id=3207>.

Trubshaw, Bob. "Paganism in British Folk Customs." *At the Edge: Exploring New Interpretations of Past and Place in Archaeology, Folklore and Mythology* 3 (1996). 14 July 2007 <http://www.indigogroup.co.uk/edge/paganism.htm>.

Wilby, Emma. *Cunning Folk and Familiar Spirits: Shamanistic Visionary Traditions in Early Modern British Witchcraft and Magic*. Brighton [UK]: Sussex Academic Press, 2005.

Winiarski, Douglas L. "Popular Belief and Expression." *Encyclopedia of American Cultural and Intellectual History*. New York: Charles's Scribner's Sons, 2001.

Younger, Lillye. "Midwifery Work Came From Necessity." 2007. *Yesterday's Tennessee*. 14 July 2007 <http://www.tnyesterday.com/books/action2/events-2.html>.

Chapter Eleven

Miranda Aldhouse-Green, and Stephen Aldhouse-Green, *The Quest of the Shaman: Shape-shifters, Sorcerers and Spirit-healers*, London: Thames & Hudson, 2005.

Chapter Twelve! (no citations)

Epilogue

Norton, Robert, and Richard Southern. *SoulTypes: Decode Your Spiritual DNA to Create a Life of Authenticity, Joy, and Grace*. San Francisco, CA: Jossey-Bass, 2004

Hirsh, Sandra Krebs, and Jane A. G. Kise. *SoulTypes: Matching Your Personality and Spiritual Path*. Minneapolis: Augsburg Books, 2006.

Appendix

Herr, Karl. *Hex and Spellwork: The Magical Practices of the Pennsylvania Dutch*. York Beach, ME: Red Wheel/Weiser, 2002.

Smith, Eliot Marshall. *The Magic Square*. 15 September 2007. <http://www.smithtrust.com/satorsite/index.html>

Stuhlman, Daniel. "Abracadabra." December 2002. *Librarian's Lobby*. 15 September 2007 <http://home.earthlink.net/~ddstuhlman/crc55.htm>

Watson, Greig. "Artefact Recalls Witches' Shadow." 28 January 2004. *BBC News*. 08 August 2007. <http://news.bbc.co.uk/1/hi/england/lincolnshire/3437241>.

Whitcombe, Chris. "Healing Stones." 1999. *Earth Mysteries*. 14 July 2007 <http://witcombe.sbc.edu/earthmysteries/EMHealing.html>.

Handsome books for a wide range of interests from **Busca**Inc

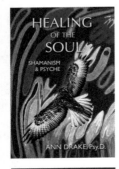

HEALING OF THE SOUL
Shamanism and Psyche
Ann Drake, Psy.D.

"One of the most detailed descriptions of shamanic healing in the literature. Drake begins with her shamanic initiations in the jungles of Borneo and takes us through her journey as a clinical psychologist dedicated to the healing of her clients. In so doing, she extends the territory of shamanism into clinical psychology by demonstrating, through clinical case histories, how shamanic techniques enhance the healing of traumatic and dissociative disorders."
—Larry Peters, PhD., The Foundation for Shamanic Studies
ISBN: 0-9666196-6-8 | 197 pages, paperback $18.95

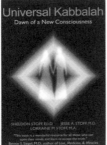

UNIVERSAL KABBALAH
Dawn of a New Consciousness
Dr. Sheldon Stoff, Jesse A. Stoff, Lorraine M. Stoff

Open to the spiritual, expand your consciousness, and go beyond the self-centered ego. Dr. Sheldon Stoff, professor emeritus at Adelphi University writes that most of us live in a cave seeing little but shadows, and offers good advice on how to get out of the cave through the four pillars of studying; praying; meditating and chanting; and doing or fulfilling Mitzvot (good deeds).
ISBN: 0-9666196-5-X | cloth $19.95

BATTLEGROUNDS OF FREEDOM
A Historical Guide to the Battlefields of the War of American Independence
Norman Desmarais

A fascinating travelogue through the battles of the Revolutionary War, Battlegrounds invites readers to vicariously re-enact each battle exactly where and how it was fought. Desmarais lays out the geographic and strategic contexts of each struggle, and develops their human dimensions with anecdotes and stories. Conveniently organized by geographic location, with references to websites, visitor centers, museums, and actual battleground sites.
ISBN: 0-9666196-7-6 | 241 pages, 64 pages of maps & photos, paperback $26.95

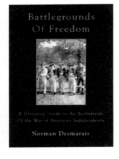

DEVIL DOGS AND JARHEADS
Victor W. Pearn

The world of the U.S. Marine in 1969 comes to life in Victor Pearn's poems of buzz cuts, reveille, drill sergeants, salutes, rifle ranges, purple hearts, sand crabs, and daily inspections. **Garrison Keillor has twice read from these pages on his NPR show *The Writer's Almanac*.**
"Victor's poetry contains both strength and appealing imagery." —Gwendolyn Brooks
"A good choice for 20th-century American poetry collections."—*American Libraries*
ISBN:0-9666196-3-3 | paperback $14.95

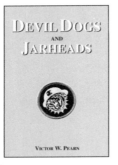

A FARM GIRL IN THE GREAT DEPRESSION
Ruth Myer

In the depths of the Great Depression many found jobs with the WPA or CCC. Most farmers chose to stay and work their farms. Ruth Myer tells the story of growing up as just such a farmer's daughter, challenged by not just the Depression, but flood and drought disasters, too. She lends a personal perspective to lessons of perserverance, thriftiness, faith, and ingenuity learned in this unique period of America history.
ISBN: 0-9666196-0-9 | 189 pages, paperback $14.95

TO ORDER: www.**busca**inc.com | 607 546 4247 *voice* 607 546 4248 *fax*